The Leadership Hike

The Leadership Hike

Shaping Primary Care Together

Amar Rughani

Joanna Bircher

With hand-drawn illustrations by Guy Rughani

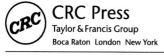

CRC Press
Taylor & Francis Group
Boca Raton London New York

CRC Press is an imprint of the
Taylor & Francis Group, an **informa** business

First edition published 2020
by CRC Press
6000 Broken Sound Parkway NW, Suite 300, Boca Raton, FL 33487-2742

and by CRC Press
2 Park Square, Milton Park, Abingdon, Oxon, OX14 4RN

© 2020 Taylor & Francis Group, LLC

First edition published by CRC Press

CRC Press is an imprint of Taylor & Francis Group, LLC

ISBN: 978-0-367-23698-4 (Paperback)
ISBN: 978-0-367-23701-1 (Hardback)
ISBN: 978-0-429-28125-9 (E-Book)

Typeset in Bembo
by Lumina Datamatics Limited

Dedication

To those who have hiked alongside us, especially our families

Contents

Forewords

This is a very significant time to be publishing a new book about leadership in primary care. Leadership matters because great care doesn't just happen. Great care is led. It requires that professionals are developed, teams are nurtured, improvement is steered, and systems change is catalysed. This new book by two inspiring primary care leaders has never been more needed.

Interest in leadership as a topic for study, discussion, research, and development has been growing in healthcare for the last 20 years or so. A generation ago leadership rarely featured in healthcare journals, conferences or professional development. The past decade has witnessed the emergence of new journals, events and courses – and more recently, leadership topics have become a regular feature in mainstream channels.

To date there has been less focus on leadership in primary care, however, and this is a trend I see not just in the UK but globally. Much of the available research, training and coaching is targeted at people working in very different environments than the average primary care team or system. There are excellent books, conferences, and courses available for healthcare leaders operating in a large corporate infrastructure, but the majority of primary care worldwide does not look like that. One can forgive primary care leaders for feeling left out.

Yet, the need for excellent leadership in primary care has never been greater, and has never had such significance for patients, the wider healthcare system and the population. The changing demographics and disease patterns we are seeing around the globe are resulting in significant growth in demand for accessible, personal, generalist care, and coordination. Patients with multiple long-term conditions do not need more specialist care but more primary care. Similarly, primary care has a crucial role as the first line of response to new problems and even pandemics.

Primary care is already responding with innovation, improvement and transformation at a pace and scale, which I don't believe we have seen before. Across the world we are seeing primary care practices expanding their teams and skill-mix, adopting innovations in access and services, incorporating more proactive and population-focused models of care, and working in closer partnership across more integrated systems of health and care.

Achieving these shifts safely, successfully, and sustainably represents a leadership challenge of unprecedented scale. The journey to realise more of our potential will require highly effective leadership of teams, of innovation and improvement, and of networks and systems. Great change doesn't just happen – it is led – and so it is high time that leadership was at the top of our agenda in primary care.

Drs Amar Rughani and Joanna Bircher are passionate about seeing primary care colleagues develop their leadership awareness, skills, and confidence. They are role models of this themselves, and have devoted themselves over the years to developing leadership effectiveness in others. This book is not just a timely reminder of the pivotal importance of leadership in meeting our challenges and opportunities – it will be an invaluable inspiration and guide as established and new leaders seek to grow themselves. I commend it to you as a treasure trove of insights to challenge and encourage you in your own leadership journey.

Dr Robert Varnam PhD MSc MRCGP
Head of General Practice Development at NHS England
GP in Rusholme, Manchester UK

Leadership is the new penicillin. Or so you might think. Leadership, if the mountain of policy documents is to be believed, is the magic bullet that will purge the National Health Service of its habitual conservatism and revitalise it with innovation, resilience, and efficiency. And if the groaning bookshelves are to be believed, there is no shortage of pundits wise enough, or self-opinionated enough, to tell us doctors how to get good at it. Leadership, apparently, is simply a matter of developing a few basic qualities – six or seven, according to Amazon's most popular books on the subject.

Those six or seven qualities (if the said popular books are to be believed) consist of vision, passion, integrity, charisma, strategic thinking, creativity, determination, communication skills, teamwork, confidence, emotional intelligence, loyalty, diplomacy, empowerment, decisiveness, focus …

Oh. We seem to have a problem. Maybe leadership isn't quite so straightforward after all.

It used to be. Back in the day, leadership just meant the bloke-in-charge telling people what to do. But because leadership is about relationships, would-be leaders found they had to temper personal power with at least a modicum of consideration for their followers. Ah, but how? Machiavelli favoured the covert approach. In his treatise of 1513, *The Prince*, he showed his royal patron how the surreptitious manipulation of underlings could pass for leadership. Machiavelli's disciples thrive to this day. Also persistently common is the 'I know best, and I'll help you see it *my* way' kind of leader. He – usually a he – is a bumptious saint, a love-child of Donald Trump and Mother Teresa, and he lives in Westminster. He has a cousin, lightweight but envious, skulking in the social media and called an 'influencer', who has nothing much to say but a compulsion to say it.

It is no criticism of leadership as a noble endeavour to say that some of its practitioners set bad examples. Such are the complexities and challenges facing the medical profession that, now more than ever, we need a better style of leadership: leadership that is not top-down or self-serving, but that comes from within; leadership that is as undemonstrative and unassertive as its results are constructive. Twenty-six centuries ago, the Taoist philosopher Lao Tzu had the right idea when he said, 'The best leader is one you hardly notice. When his work is done and his aim fulfilled, people say, *"Amazing! We did it all by ourselves"'*.

Do doctors make good leaders? Or followers, for that matter? On one hand, our medical training conditions us to believe we know what's good for other people. On the other hand, there's no reason to suppose that leadership potential can be assumed in members of a profession selected mainly for their ability as teenagers to pass exams in physics and chemistry. On the third hand, the GP consultation, in which we take such pride, is an exercise in leadership so subtle that, on a good day, it can go almost unnoticed. I suspect that most of us are quite ambivalent about leading and being led. We follow guidelines with passable grace, and can act supportive of innovations in whose creation we are told we have had a formative say. But, truth to tell, isn't there a bit of us that likes to dig our heels in? Aren't we really like the proverbial cats being herded; and don't we sometimes take a perverse pride in the comparison, and in the independence of spirit we think it represents? So who in their right mind – whether voluntarily or reluctantly – would seek or accept a leadership role in general practice?

Actually, all of us. Leadership doesn't have to be high profile, high visibility, high risk. Good leadership is arguably most valuable when it is local and low key. For every committee chairmanship there are a thousand opportunities to make things better: in the practice, at the partners' meeting, in the staff room, in the community … Look around you; you know where they are.

To paraphrase Shakespeare's famous lines, 'Be not afraid of leadership: some are born leaders, some achieve leadership, and some have leadership thrust upon them'. To the first (mercifully small) group who see themselves as natural leaders, I would say only that they may not be quite so born to it as they might suppose. They should read this book, and do a reality check.

But the authors are really speaking to the second and third groups: to those who, for the best of motives, want to contribute to the success and well-being of their colleagues, and to those who find themselves stepping up to the plate either because it's Buggins' turn or because no one else will do it. If any of these are you, take heart. This book, like general practice itself, is wide-ranging in its scope and understanding, and revelatory in the depths which it explores. It will hold your nose to the grindstone of self-examination, which is sometimes painful but is ultimately the best guarantor of insight and motivation. In it you will find no platitudes, no pious exhortations to impossible virtues. It's as nutritious and comforting as hot chocolate – and you deserve it.

Roger Neighbour OBE MA DSc FRCGP FRCP
Past President, Royal College of General Practitioners

Preface

The most important qualification for a leader is not wanting to be a leader.

Plato

So, what is leadership? It is not a role so much as what we, perhaps to our surprise, find ourselves doing. Like the canary in the coal mine, leaders notice the early need to change, and feel driven to sing out to make others move. But we are more than an alarm. To us as authors, leadership is the art of understanding influence and using it well to facilitate not just change, but also adaptation and survival. When driven by what we care about, applied through our skills and nurtured by our values, it becomes powerfully useful to our communities and facilitates everything from small improvements to radical changes in direction.

Most people want the world and the communities they care about, to be better than they are. Our simple but clear understanding is that we are only better, together, and that we make a difference through helping *others* to make a difference.

We describe that possibility, which is there within us all, drawing on our lives and our work as general medical practitioners (GPs) in the British National Health Service (NHS), where our leadership insight has been most developed.

This guide is written for all those, at whatever level in their organisation and at whatever stage of life experience, who wish to improve their ability to lead well. Because organisations are not just structures but the *people* they comprise, improving the positive influence of the individuals will collectively improve the useful influence of the organisation they are part of. This book is therefore as much about being a better practice as being a better leader.

Although we are limited by our experience, we are less so by our vision, which is of leadership that helps healthcare communities to transform well-being, not by controlling anyone, but by engaging the strengths of others. This takes place within the wider potential of leadership, which is to challenge and support people to grow, to care for those who are vulnerable and to treat our natural world with as much repect as we should show each other.

Metaphors are all around. Both of us live and work near the Peak District of England and enjoy walking in the glorious countryside, especially in company where we share a journey that over time, enriches and changes us. Leadership can't be taught, but like a hike, we can appreciate what it has to reveal much better by using our walking boots than by just looking at our maps.

This is what we seek to do. We will be your companions on the leadership hike and on the journey to come, we will describe what we see and what might be made of it. Although we can't hear your voice in this dialogue, we know it is there and because of the journey you have chosen to take, that it is growing stronger.

Amar Rughani

Joanna Bircher

Acknowledgements

There are many who have helped us to gain a better understanding of leadership, in particular our colleagues from the Chapelgreen Practice, Sheffield, and the Lockside Medical Centre, Stalybridge. We wish to thank them for supporting us to become better leaders and team members. In addition, there are many who have willingly given their time and shared their insights and experience. It would be unfair to single out any individual, but their guidance and encouragement are deeply appreciated.

Authors

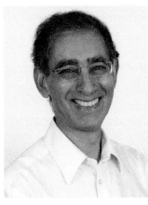

Amar Rughani
As so often in life, we neither earn nor possibly deserve some of the most significant things that come our way. I was lucky enough to be brought up with an Eastern philosophy applied in early years to a Geordie environment and to be one of a family whose diversity and encouragement remain its greatest strengths. Allied to that, I've worked with many people who see the world differently and from whom I have learned so much, my co-author Joanna being a notable example.

People are at the heart of this and it seemed natural and meaningful to become a GP, the medical vocation that most strongly encouraged me to appreciate those I served not as patients with conditions, but as real people living real lives.

To understand people is to understand leadership. It's not leaders who make the difference and Lincoln had it right when in one of the most inspiring speeches in history, he talked of better lives being created 'by the people, for the people'. Although I've held a number of positions that granted me the power and the expectation of authority, my most profound understanding of leadership has come about despite, and not because, of them.

If I have any qualification to write on the subject, it is that I care about people, am amazed at what we are capable of at our best, and believe in the fertility of collaboration over the impotence of domination. Many are similarly qualified and because of this, we are as much your fellow travellers as your guides on the leadership hike.

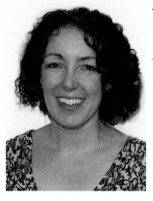

Joanna Bircher

Since qualifying as a GP in 1999, I have been given many opportunities to expand my day job beyond the consultation room. I have been an appraiser, an appraisal lead, a mentor, and coach. I have experienced leadership at many levels; in my practice, in a Commissioning Group, across Greater Manchester and at a national level with the Royal College of GPs. Every opportunity has been a chance to learn new things and has stretched me in ways I couldn't have predicted.

Though the roles have been varied, each one has helped me to explore leadership, both by observing others in this role and by trying things out myself. I have come to know the power of people to make great things happen if they are in the right environment and given the right support. This power seems to come from the strength of connection between people and their belief in their ability to make a difference.

Contributing to this book was my opportunity to share this learning, and for readers to see if it connects with their own experience. It may be that not everything will resonate with you, but my hope is that it will help you to gain insights that might help you on your own leadership hike.

Our landscape: The complex world in which we work and lead

Section introduction

Although most of this book encourages us to think deeply about ourselves and how we can best influence the world around us, this section starts somewhere else entirely. Before we start with ourselves, we want to spend some time looking outwardly; before any journey it is vital to understand the terrain that we are navigating. This terrain has several aspects. It includes the context in which we work, both at the level of our organisation and more widely, including what may be happening in our local area as well as nationally and internationally. These factors often have direct impact on the influence we have.

Ideas around effective leadership change over time and depend on context. Individuals, who have been held in high regard in the past for their leadership skills, may now be seen as autocratic and oppressive. Understanding the current thinking around effective leadership in healthcare helps us to see how we fit in, and to understand that effective leaders don't have to be born with natural leadership traits but develop these over time.

Our experience of leading, and helping others to do so, has told us, time after time, of the importance of the circumstances that surround us to the end result of our actions. We have found that what works in one setting, with one group of people, then doesn't work with another. This isn't a recipe for disillusionment; far from it, because it is the nature of the world that it can be shaped but not controlled, by us. We can therefore, with realism, aspire to adapting to the world with agility, our shoulders free of the weight of expectation that the future is in our hands.

1

Context and organisational culture and how to influence it

In this chapter, we will explore these questions:

- How can we better understand the context in which we are working?
- How can we lead when there are so many factors that appear to be out with our control?
- What is organisational culture, how does it develop and is there anything we can do to shift it?
- Aren't some problems just too hard to solve?

What do we mean by context?

One of the best analogies on context we have read comes from Binnie et al.'s book *Living Leadership*. They talk about the role of the weather for a sailor trying to navigate from one place to the next. The weather is the context. They don't complain about the weather, or deny its significance. In fact, an understanding of the weather and how to adapt to it is crucial to the success of their journey. They don't see the weather as the 'problem' and them as the 'answer', and recognise that, even if they make predictions, these may turn out to be wrong and they will need to adapt, and even, at times, make little progress on their journey until the conditions improve.

Context is a very broad term that includes factors as wide-ranging as changes in government, to the culture of the organisation where we work. It's sometimes difficult to predict how a contextual issue will make a difference to outcome. In this chapter we start from the wider concept, looking at the health system as a whole and then narrow down to our local systems and then down to our organisation, looking specifically at culture, how to assess it and how we might influence it.

The health service as a complex adaptive system

Experts in organisational theory suggest that our healthcare context can be thought of as a *complex adaptive system*. We will consider the system first and then the implications for leadership.

Complex adaptive systems consist of a large number of elements, in this case organisations of varying sizes, which interact, with any element in the system being affected by, and affecting, several other systems. The interactions between the elements are often not linear, with individuals interacting with different elements simultaneously. Elements in the system are often not aware of what is happening in other parts of the system, nor are they aware of the whole system behaviour and tend to respond only to what they can see happening nearby. Present behaviour of elements in the system has been shaped by history, and not all elements have experienced the same influences.

The system includes any one of the millions of the population who may, usually unpredictably, interact with the system at any time. This means the system is 'open', as it is difficult to define the boundaries. The system operates within a social, political, financial and technological landscape that is also constantly changing, and yet changes in these can influence the ability of the healthcare system to deliver care to the population it serves.

As a way of illustrating the interdependencies of a complex adaptive system, let's look at a 23-year-old presenting in primary care with symptoms of generalised anxiety.

His decision whether to present his symptoms to a GP in the first place will be influenced by pre-existing beliefs about mental health and illness, which will have been influenced by the experience and attitudes of family members and peers as well as social attitudes and social media. It may also have been influenced by previous experience of the GP practice and the ease of access to an appointment.

What takes place during the consultation will be influenced by the GP's experience, both professionally and personally, of mental health, as well as by the current advice on management by experts who provide guidance. It may have been influenced, even unwittingly, by the GP's exposure to pharmaceutical advertising.

Factors influencing the action planned may include the availability of psychological therapy, including the availability of voluntary/third-sector provision, which varies geographically. The availability will have been influenced by the priorities of the organisation that commissions the service, and by the changes in demand for the service. Changes in demand will have been influenced by changes in societal attitudes as well as economic factors resulting in more triggers to poor mental health such as unemployment and poverty.

The commissioning organisations' priorities and the amount invested in services for people with anxiety symptoms will have been influenced by national priorities, which in turn can be influenced by societal attitudes and media campaigns or pressure groups. The total funds available to spend on any aspect of health care will be influenced by the changing demographic, with money being needed to support the ageing population with increasing morbidity and long-term conditions such as diabetes and heart disease. Many of these conditions are lifestyle-driven and therefore influenced by the ease of access to cheap unhealthy food and the reduced opportunities for exercise.

The system is clearly complex, but it is also adaptive. It changes in response to the changes that occur in the elements within it and to the external factors that interact with it. A true complex adaptive system is self-organising with no hierarchy of command, adapting and learning to create a best fit with the surrounding environment. In our health service, the 'best fit' is not always the end result, as some stakeholders hold more power to influence the system than others and the voice of the patient or the smaller elements can sometimes be lost.

What are the implications for leadership? The system may seem self-organising, but we are not powerless to have a useful influence on the emerging changes. The system is not just the structure but also the people, and when we think about the system adapting to changes, we particularly mean that the people, and notably the leaders, have to be adaptable. To be effective leaders we need to be alert with respect to changes to context and spot opportunities for influence. We need a flexible mindset to be open to the ideas of others, free enough to abandon what isn't working and move on and energetic enough to do so quickly.

A GP practice as a complex adaptive system

It's not just the wider context that is complex. Our GP practices and local networks can also be viewed as complex adaptive systems that respond to internal and external influences in ways that may be unpredictable. The diagram shown here illustrates just a few of the complex factors affecting general practice in recent years including some of the adaptations that have resulted; we're sure you can think of many more.

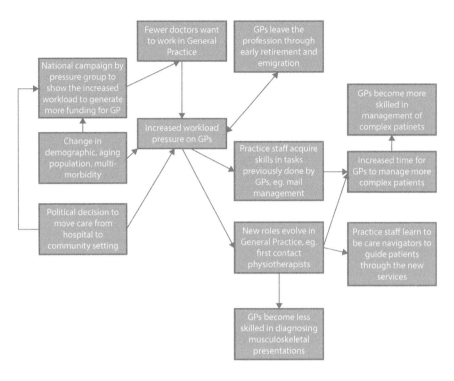

The adaptations have required not only the development of skills but also shifts in attitudes related to power, safety, whose job it is and how to communicate changes to our patients. There is often lack of certainty as to whether the response/adaptation is the right one, especially as some of the adaptations can bring harm as well as benefit. Our role as leaders is to maintain confidence through the uncertainty and observe and respond to what arises during the adaptation.

Organisational culture

One of the most important aspects of the immediate context where we work is the organisation culture. This is something that will have developed over years and is seen in the habits and behaviours that happen day to day. Simply put, it is 'the way we do things round here'. When you are deeply embedded within an organisation it can be very hard to identify the culture, although often it is easy to see the impact.

The NHS has a number of cultural features which include having a 'not-for-profit' ethos, an appropriate concern for patient safety that can extend risk-aversion to non-clinical areas, and being insulated from the commercial marketplace and the pressure to compete.

Management consultant Peter Drucker once famously stated, 'Culture eats strategy for breakfast'; whether our great plans are actually implemented will depend on the values, assumptions and behaviours of those with whom we work. In Chapter 10, we will be looking at power and influence. Who holds power, and how, are important elements of the culture of our organisations.

New members of the team, including temporary workers such as trainees or apprentices, will soon work out the culture and adapt to it. Within a short space of time they are likely to have acquired the same habits and may only appreciate the impact of that culture when they move to a different organisation.

It might be helpful to use a framework to analyse the culture of our organisation, describing three levels: what we see around us, what we value and what assumptions we make.

What we see around us	These are the things that can be easily seen or heard, and include our rituals and routines, for example: • *How people address each other?* • *What types of things are talked about at break times?* • *Where people leave their bags, coats, etc.?* • *What can be seen on the walls?* • *How often GPs leave their consultation room?* • *Who makes the tea/coffee?* • *Who washes up/loads the dishwasher?* • *How people communicate urgent tasks?* • *Who usually responds to urgent communications?* • *What the response is to a GP/nurse running late?* • *How we deal with patients who are late for appointments?* • *How we respond to staff errors?* • *Do meetings always start late? Does anyone mind?*
What everyone values	Examples of values: • *We value people over process* • *We value safety over innovation* • *We value hierarchy and order* • *We value high-quality clinical performance* • *We value top financial performance* • *We value tidiness/promptness*

(Continued)

7

What assumptions we make	These are largely unconscious but underlie the other aspects of culture. Examples of assumptions: • *We assume everyone is trying their hardest so if an error occurs, we need to look at factors that led to the error, rather than find someone to blame* • *We assume everyone has the capacity to learn 'on the job' and so encourage staff to take on extra roles without specific training* • *We assume people will be lazy if allowed to be, so will divide out tasks evenly so that it is fair* • *We assume GPs are more important members of the team and so will allocate them a specific parking space* • *Being prompt to a meeting means people care about the organisation*

Because assumptions are implicit, we as leaders don't always recognise the effects they have on behaviour. For example, practices that allocate specific parking spaces for GPs because of historic practice might not have seen how this reinforces a hierarchy that has impeded other team members from taking responsibility for new roles. Practices that eat lunch together, sharing stories from their home life, may not have recognised that it was these conversations that resulted in a culture of team members caring for each other and staff being prepared to work extra shifts to cover colleagues when they are sick.

As leaders, our actions can sometimes have an impact on culture that we didn't intend, sometimes with harmful consequences. For example, a new GP partner may have led a change in managing the GP visit allocation to ensure that the visits are distributed fairly. Previously, the culture was more collaborative, with GPs volunteering to visit the patients they knew best and those with fewer administrative responsibilities in the practices doing more visits. The new system drove the partnership to think about distributing other tasks more equally, but this resulted in a new priority given to 'fairness' over the collaborative culture that had existed previously. This resulted in higher levels of work stress, and doctors being less inclined to 'step in' to help out colleagues who were running late.

As leaders, the actions we take can either reinforce old culture or can be part of shifting to new patterns. This can sometimes cause disruption and temporary disharmony. A practice manager who valued tidiness had become aware of a culture of disorganisation and untidiness at their practice was resulting in things getting lost, with time being wasted trying to find things. The practice decided they would work on this, although not everyone was yet on board with the idea. The PM decided to clear the 'clutter' from the practice nurse's room whilst she was on holiday as what he thought was a favour to her. Unfortunately, the act had unintended consequences as the nurse cared deeply about some of the items that had been discarded. She interpreted the act as the PM undervaluing her as a team member. This is not to say the act was wrong, just that we need to avoid assumptions, create opportunities to have conversations about our intended actions and uncover the consequences that these might have.

Assessing and measuring organisational culture is no easy task. There have been a number of publications related to questionnaires that can be used to assess whether our practice has a 'safety culture', one of which, **Safequest**, has been widely used in practice. These questionnaires are based on the recognition that excessive workload, poor communication, rigid hierarchy, punitive action/blame after error, inconsistent processes and poor teamwork will result in a climate detrimental to patient safety. They may be a useful starting point to assess practice culture.

Just stopping to think about it, however, might be the most useful thing we can do. This is especially useful to do in conversation with someone who may have joined the practice from elsewhere. Finding out what they have noticed, and then thinking about how this may reflect underlying values and assumptions, gives us a starting point to assess where we are, and where we might prefer to be.

Shifting organisational culture

Shifting the culture of organisations is one of the hardest tasks of a leader, often because the assumptions underlying the culture are hidden to all, including the leader. Shifting culture takes time, because developing the culture took time. At times it can be useful to create or identify a disturbance that is big enough for people to accept a need for change. However, we should be careful before trying this, as generating anxiety that results in people becoming fearful of taking action could itself become the new culture we embed.

The GP who was trying to develop a new culture of tidiness might use the fact that something very important or very expensive had gone missing as a way of encouraging others to place a higher value on tidiness. In Chapter 23, we introduce Kotter's stages of change management. Generating a disturbance like this would be Kotter's 'creating a burning platform' to trigger change. Although disturbance can be useful, it needs to be balanced with a feeling of hope, with opportunity for people to generate creative solutions.

Changing the nature of the conversations that take place in the practice can be a slow but very effective way of shifting culture. This can also involve creating the opportunity for these conversations to occur by ensuring that there is time and space and that meeting agendas are not so full of tasks and business that effective dialogue never takes place (see Chapter 9). Unless we view conversations as being effective ways of making change happen, we won't value them. If we don't value them then we will always be too busy to have them. As a leader, we should welcome such conversations and try to master the art of not looking too busy to have them, even if it feels like there are always more pressing things to do. In these conversations, we pay attention to the ideas that promote the culture we want to develop and encourage and celebrate moves in the right direction, however small they may appear.

Sometimes doing something 'symbolic' to indicate the shift in culture we are aiming for can be helpful. Buying a fancy coffee machine for staff can demonstrate we value them as people, not just as staff; starting up new rituals such as an extra day's leave on team members' birthdays can have a similar outcome. However, even symbolic gestures like this can backfire if the current culture is far from where we want it to be. Introducing a 'day off on your birthday' becomes fraught if staff start complaining it is unfair when their birthday falls at a weekend.

Once we clarify our current culture and the shifts we want to make, we can use this when selecting new members of the team, particularly looking out for those that embody the desired values. It doesn't take long, however, for new team members to acquire the habits they see around them, especially if they don't feel they have the power to comment or influence. New team members who frequently comment, 'When I worked at the other place we used to …' are not always treated warmly if feedback is perceived as criticism. However, handled carefully, and if the existing team know new people have been asked to come up with ideas that might help everyone, this can be a useful intervention.

Our own behaviours can be powerful signals of the change we want to see and can help to change the behaviour of others. For example, one practice used to use a loudspeaker to call in patients for their appointments. One of their GP Specialty Trainees didn't like the loudspeaker and preferred to walk into the waiting room to fetch their patients. The trainee used the opportunity to connect with the patients, and made the wait less stressful for those with hearing impairment or those who may have felt anxious about missing their name when called. The trainee also liked being less sedentary. Conversations were had about his way of doing things. The GP partners and practice nurses held shared values but hadn't recognised the impact of the loudspeaker on patients or their own health. The behaviour rubbed off and after 6 months no one was using the old call-in system.

Organisational culture in new organisations and networks

Recent developments in primary care, particularly in the United Kingdom, have focused on better collaboration between practices that are working in a defined locality. In some of these networks, a wide range of organisations attempt to deliver some services together, often from a background of different cultures. If it is a challenge for us to understand and influence the culture of our own organisation, imagine the challenge of scaling this up.

In this scenario there is an opportunity to develop a new overarching culture for the network, as long as we start by establishing a shared set of values that will underpin what we deliver (see Chapter 25). Leading a network of practices in the process of establishing these values seems like a huge task and large sums of money could be paid to consultancy firms to make this happen. We suggest that this isn't needed. Instead, we could focus on the art of conversation (see Chapter 9), creating time and space to listen and be heard. This means not relying on email as a way of communicating ideas. Transmitting information by email has become embedded as the main route for communicating across more health services due to its convenience, to the detriment of effective dialogue. Via email, nuances can't be heard; there is no opportunity for non-verbal cues to be delivered or received and shared values can't be established.

In response to the challenges of increasing demand for care and a reduction in available workforce, many practices are choosing to merge to become a single organisation. In our experience, much attention is paid to the practicalities and the logistics of staff employment, buildings, IT systems, telephones and timetables and too little attention paid to the huge challenge of identifying and merging organisations with different cultures. However, this is every bit as important as the logistics if we are to retain a happy, thriving workforce.

Think about:

- What rituals exist in each practice (e.g. around birthdays, festivals such as Christmas, breaktimes), and how to capture the best of all of them
- Where the power lies in each practice
- What symbols of hierarchy exists (uniforms, parking spaces, forms of address) and how can these be merged if they are very different
- What the 'stories', their history and key events that need to be celebrated and shared with the others are for each practice

There isn't a perfect 'blueprint' on how to do this, but just recognising it as an issue that needs to be managed is a very good start.

Dealing with complexity and solving 'wicked' problems

At the start of this chapter we talked about the health service as a complex adaptive system and described various levels of complexity.

If we are developing new services, or improving existing ones, we need to be aware of the context that we are working within. If we think the change is linear and that there may be a simple solution, we are probably wrong. However, complex is not the same as chaotic. Stacey's grid is often used to explain complexity, and this is shown in the diagram that follows.

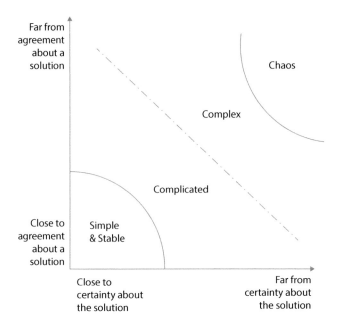

The graph shows the relationship between how certain we are about the behaviour of our system, or the solution we have chosen for our problem and how much agreement there is between all parties about the solution. The further away we are from certainty about the solution and from agreement with others, the more we move from a 'simple' zone through the complicated zone and into a complex one. As leaders we are tasked with keeping our organisations out of 'chaos' as this is a precarious and unstable state.

Complicated problems differ from complex (sometimes known as 'wicked') problems. In a complicated problem it is possible to know the answer, even though multiple factors might need to be considered and multiple steps carried out. Despite the multiple factors, each one is known and predictable and therefore a perfect (or near-perfect) solution is theoretically possible.

To illustrate the concept, we will consider three different scenarios related to the annual practice influenza immunisation campaign:

1 **Simple problem** – Running out of flu jabs before the end of the season.
   In this scenario, all were agreed that the reason they had run out was because they had failed to recognise the increasing list size of the practice and had used the previous year's order for vaccines to guide how many were ordered this year. Everyone agreed that the following year they would renew the search on the number of eligible patients and calculate the order based in this.

2 **Complicated** – Organising rooms and staff availability to run the flu clinics.
   Although this can be complicated, we know the number of staff we have, the hours they work, the number of rooms available and the number of vaccines that need to be given. It may take lots of thinking and planning to get to the solution, but a solution that is very likely to work is at least possible.

3 **Complex** – How to increase our uptake of flu jabs by the at-risk populations.
   In this situation there are more unpredictable factors at play, and elements in the system we can't influence. It may depend on the press reports on the efficacy of last year's vaccine or social media output from people against vaccination. It could also be influenced by the weather, or by early flu outbreaks that could improve uptake. We might try different call-up methods without knowing in advance which would be more effective.

Leadership is a function of what we do, not what role we have. Recognising this can free people from traditional leadership hierarchies. In the example given, we might imagine that it isn't the nominal leaders of the practice that work through the complex issue of increasing flu immunisation uptake, but a small group led, for example, by the patient participation group.

Each type of problem requires a different leadership approach and different skills.

Leaders work with problems on a continuum from simple to complex. Problems are not uniform and complex problems can have simple parts. We need leadership at every level, but we pull on more of our leadership skills when the issues are complex because it is in this area that people most need to be involved rather than controlled.

Complicated problems may have many elements and at first sight look overwhelming, but the elements can be identified and their relationship with each other understood well enough that we can predict what would happen to 'B' if we made a stipulated change to 'A'. In this situation, we can devise an intervention, plan what we propose to do and look for the predicted outcome.

In complex contexts, this doesn't apply. The lack of predictability means that these situations can't be treated as technical problems which can be solved through known methods. The mindset needed is not of an expert, solving a difficult problem, but of an experimenter who knows that a way forward can be found through trial and learning. Anxiety and fear, which can undermine progress, can be reduced by confidence in such an attitude and an approach. For all of these reasons, complex problems need adaptive approaches with leaders who are able to be agile and recognise that whereas technical problems can be solved, complex problems have to be worked through. A good outcome from such leadership is that the team become more adaptable and that today's complex issues become tomorrow's technical problems.

Over the stile

Having explored the complex landscape of health care, and the multiple factors affecting how much we are able to influence outcomes, it is possible we feel powerless to make meaningful change. If we have 'stepped up' to lead it can take time to work out what we need to do to be effective in this new role. In the next chapter we will look at the changing view of leadership in the modern age and how this might mean rejecting some of our pre-conceived ideas about how leaders should think and behave.

Bibliography

Bate, P. (2014). *Context Is Everything: In Perspectives in Context.* London, UK: The Health Foundation. Available at http://health.org.uk/publications/perspectives-on-context/.

Binney, G., Wilke, G., & Williams, C. (2005). *Living Leadership: A Practical Guide for Ordinary Heroes.* London, UK: Prentice Hall.

Grint, K. (2005). Problems, problems, problems: The social construction of leadership. *Human Relations* 58(11), 1467–1494.

Health Improvement Scotland. (2012). Safequest safety climate survey. Available at www.healthcareimprovementscotland.org/our_work/patient_safety/spsp_primary_care_resources/safety_climate_survey.aspx.

Heifetz, R., Grashow, A., & Linsky, M. (2009). *The Practice of Adaptive Leadership.* Harvard Business Review Press. ISBN 978-14221-0576-4.

Schein, E.H. (2010). *Organizational Culture and Leadership* (4th ed.). San Francisco, CA: Jossey-Bass.

Stacey. R. (2012). *The Tools and Techniques of Leadership and Management: Meeting the Challenge of Complexity.* London, UK: Routledge.

2

Perspectives on leadership

In this chapter, we will explore these questions:

- What are the expectations made of modern leaders and how do these compare to the past?
- Why is understanding ourselves so important and how does this relate to our influence?
- Primary care gives potential leaders a running start. Why is this?
- Are management and leadership at odds with each other?

A historical perspective

Effective leadership depends on the context, which includes the era in which it is practised. What was suited to the past is not suited to the present and, despite what we might hope, what we recommend in this book may not suit in perpetuity. When we think about leadership, we don't start with a clean slate. Everyone has a view and our biases and assumptions come from leadership's historical context, which we will now briefly consider.

The literature on leadership is vast, reflecting both the perennial interest in the subject and the often unreasonable weight of expectation that society has placed on what leadership is capable of. There have been trends in thinking, which have included the 'great man' theory of leadership from the nineteenth century, postulating that certain inborn character traits such as charisma and intellect made people (men) suited for leadership, such people often being characterised as heroic figures. However, subsequent research has not confirmed that traits reliably distinguish between leaders and non-leaders.

In the twentieth century we had the idea of 'transformational leadership' in which, as Bernard Bass describes it, 'leaders broaden and elevate the interests of their employees, when they generate awareness and acceptance of the purposes and mission of the group, and when they stir their employees to look beyond their own self-interest for the good of the group'.

These attributes remain important. In later thinking, reflecting a growing appreciation of complexity and chaos, authors have seen leadership as relating to the ability to be 'catalysts for complex, emergent change within interactive networks, of which they form a part'.

In the twenty-first century, we have seen a number of notable examples, particularly in the political world, of leaders who have broken the mould of possessing the traditionally expected virtues. Such people have not been notable for altruism, integrity or even honesty, but have nevertheless been elected, even re-elected, and have been associated with change, partly through disruption. However, health care, which is deeply values-based and where integrity and trust matter, may be a different story regarding the attributes required of its leaders.

Nevertheless, whatever the values different communities in society require from their leaders, these have to be applied in a world that is complex and swampy. In such a world, the problems we manage are rarely simple ones where technical solutions will suffice. The way forward cannot be predetermined, because it doesn't reside in experts or leaders but instead in the collective thinking and application of our team. Our role as leaders is therefore to *involve* people rather than instruct them.

In more recent times, a powerful body of evidence has shown that in the health service, a more collective form of leadership that engages people's initiative, drive and skills, is much more effective in improving outcomes at all levels. This is called 'compassionate leadership' and because it's about *engaging* people, the concept is much broader and tougher than being 'nice'; its principles, as articulated by Michael West, resonate strongly with the mindset we adopt in this book.

So where is leadership going? Don Berwick, reflecting on the history of health care, has talked of a third era in which we move beyond the unassailable professions of era one and the target-driven measurement culture of era two, into an age where leadership creates the culture that humane health care needs. In the coming age, he emphasises the importance of civility and transparency. As a renowned expert in health care improvement, he talks of the importance of performance being driven by science, namely quality improvement rather than by ideology. Importantly, he reminds us as leaders that the best health care arises when we listen closely and work for patients as their servants rather than turn a deaf ear and seek to control them as their masters.

As leaders in the modern age, we have a particularly difficult challenge. The historic command and control structure and traditional leadership expectations of primary care teams are still strong but they are not suited to the collective way in which teams must now work in order to thrive. Developing the team to become more empowered and capable will not be easy; it may not even be welcomed, but it is necessary and our task will be leading the cultural change that makes that happen. That change must begin with ourselves.

The difficulties in making cultural change will not just be with our own teams; this is because we will connect increasingly with other organisations that influence our work. Many of these will be top-down hierarchies and the culture clash will be painful. Nevertheless, because our collective work will be more empowering, more productive and will lead to greater well-being, it is a challenge worth rising to.

Being a leader

As we journey together in this book, we will develop a much greater understanding of ourselves and of how we apply that understanding to develop an effective team, but why is this important?

Leadership is a people – and in our context, a relationship – ability. Primarily, it's there to help communities to move forward in a world in which, as we've established, we face problems that are complex rather than 'just' complicated.

People move forward, and if we get it wrong, backward, by influencing each other and leaders have a particular need and responsibility to influence well. This we do by understanding our *actual* influence (how we are affecting others) and our *best* influence, which comes from appreciating our genuine selves. This is not a philosophical exercise alone but a practical one, because the better we understand and use our dispositions and our strengths, the better we can help people and the more strongly they may wish to collaborate.

The journey to understanding and being our best selves is as tough as it is worthwhile. We have to recognise and peel back our façades, which include the roles and identities that we have accepted, such as parent, child, partner and professional. Although strong and often laudable, these façades project some aspects of ourselves but obscure the more complete person within. They are important and necessary but, whilst living these personae, we must learn to see through them so that we can appreciate our more complete selves and thereby understand our motivations, values, dispositions and strengths. These are the deeper things that people connect to and are helped by, more strongly than by any façade.

As we become more aware of what we are, we can help that self to be more powerfully expressed through the identities that we inhabit in the real world. In this way, the best of what we have to give is liberated. The process goes beyond ourselves, because as we learn to 'give birth to ourselves', as Erich Fromm memorably put it, we can help others in our community to do likewise.

Applying ourselves so that we help each other more humanely and effectively takes great but not unattainable skill. Working in primary care gives us a significant advantage because we are used to building effective trusting relationships that give people confidence to move forward despite complexity and uncertainty. If we can combine these skills with the ability to tailor our influence well, we can be great leaders. This does not mean great in the egotistical sense, but in terms of the great capability we can foster in our communities.

The evidence shows that our communities, working as task-orientated teams, will be successful if the following conditions are met:

- The team must be cared about.
- They must be engaged in work that is meaningful to them.
- They must have a few clear goals.
- They must be well-led.

The rest of this book will illuminate how we do this.

Change and the roles of leaders and managers

You manage things; you lead people.

Grace Hopper

How communities move forward, as we discuss further in Chapter 24, requires an appreciation of change. Change is continual and how we adapt and evolve successfully through it is the business of leaders. However, it is also the work of managers, so how are the two roles related?

As we have noted, leadership is a people skill and is needed in situations where control is not possible or appropriate, for example:

- When we need to question, 'Are we doing the *right thing*, rather than doing *things right*?'
- When the problem can't be sorted with a technical fix but requires us to *adapt*.
- When we need people's *engagement* to generate ideas or attempt different ways of doing things, not just their *effort*.

Management, on the other hand, will exercise control and will usually do so legitimately. In situations that are better understood and less unstable, managers bring order and predictability and are therefore invaluable when planning, organising, implementing and evaluating are needed.

Leaders come into their own when situations are less certain or stable. We help people to imagine possibilities, decide on direction, experiment with change and generate the motivation to move into the future with purpose. Through this process, parts of a complex issue, like improving access, crystallise out into 'fixes' like care navigation which can be designed and implemented. As they do so, these become the province of managers, allowing leaders to keep engaging with complexity, which is where our expertise is best applied. In real life, though, how often does that happen?

The mindsets of leaders and managers are both complementary and appropriately different. Leaders are expected to be bold and they encourage thinking and action that bring risk because their outcomes are unknown. Managers, on the other hand, will try to stabilise situations and reduce the risk that comes from disturbance to the system.

Managers and leaders are often contrasted in books on leadership in negative ways that suggest that management is a stultifying activity that not only maintains the status quo but also is antipathetic to the goals of leadership. We believe this to be unfair, as managers are as much a part of the process of successful change as those whose strengths in facilitating change lie in different areas.

There is also no rank order to the difficulty of the work of leaders as compared to that of managers. Even though the work of leaders can be high-profile and high-stakes, the everyday life of managers has been characterised as 'hectic, varied, fragmented, reactive, disorderly and political', i.e. every bit as challenging.

Leaders need management skills and, just as importantly, managers need leadership skills. Why? For leaders to delegate management entirely to managers is unreasonable and denies us the opportunity to learn from the nitty-gritty of implementing change in ways that would enhance our ability to help teams work effectively.

Likewise, if managers absent themselves from using leadership skills, they might be tempted to push through changes that they knew were not working rather than pause and use a leadership mindset to ask questions, get people on board and possibly change tack. Both leaders and managers become more agile and effective by sharing, rather than delegating, each other's skills and responsibilities.

So, in brief, taking the organisation forward is about getting things done. The vision that leadership generates is brought into being and sustained through good management. The achievements resulting from good management further promote effective leadership. Both are needed in order to progress.

Having now discussed the context of leadership, we will move forward and explore how change begins at home, namely with ourselves.

2

Ourselves:
Knowing me …

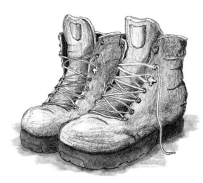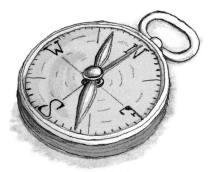

Section introduction

We have surveyed the terrain and established some major principles for effective leadership in primary care. No successful hike is possible without our walking boots to get a confident grip, and a compass to give us a sense of direction. In leadership terms, our walking boots represent our influence and our compass signifies what we care about and feel we must move toward. Both are essential, because we need them throughout our journey.

Let's keep it simple.

We become effective leaders because we really *care about something* that also matters to others. They collaborate with us because they know that we really *care about them*.

This section is about ourselves, our personal influence and how we cultivate that in order to help people. So that we don't get lost in the detail, it's helpful to describe the bigger picture as we see it. To become effective leaders we:

- *Use our energy and drive.* We recognise when something needs to change, and care about it enough to initiate moves in that direction. We feel for where the energy lies in ourselves and in the community and learn to channel that energy so that it flows in a direction that helps us all. We use our drive to keep others sufficiently energised, a process that requires our persistence, determination and at times, courage.

- *Continually try to become our best selves,* because this is where our most useful influence comes from. In broad terms, we try to live with integrity and use the strengths of our values, attitudes and skills. Because we can only move forward by collaborating with each other, we need the strengths of others to complement our own. Therefore, helping others to be their best selves becomes as important as nurturing that in ourselves.

- *Care about others and behave with kindness,* which means that in addition to caring for ourselves, we learn to respect others, reduce the status gap between us and help people to give their best. We do this in ways that are encouraging, persistent and humane. Through this we become less self-orientated and more concerned for others, both because it is ethical to be so and because it is needed to help us all to move forward.

As we discover more about ourselves and our influence, we learn to use it so that we might help others better and do more good, but equally importantly, do less harm.

As authors we don't claim to be experts, just experienced practitioners. Hands up, we've made many mistakes along the way and gone off in the wrong direction many a time. However, that's how we learn and as a result we've picked up some thoughts, not tips, about how to use our influence better and it is these that we will share.

How to share these is problematic, because the topic of how people relate to each other and try to collaborate is vast. It would be impossible to cover everything, and it would also be presumptuous to claim that we have identified the most important elements. So instead what we have chosen to do is to say 'This is a puzzle; we can see and understand some of the pieces but there may be others, perhaps known to you rather than to us, that are missing'.

In this section, we describe five pieces of the jigsaw and our hope is that you will accept them for what they are and use them to reflect on, challenge their validity and make some sense of them in the context of your own journey.

You can read this section in one go, that's up to you, but we suggest that you come back to it as you continue your journey, and use the bigger picture described above so that you can see the wood as well as the trees. As you do so, you will gain greater insight as you link the ideas to later sections on team-working, and at the end of the book, thoughts on leadership at wider levels of influence.

To give you an overview of this section of our leadership hike, here are the pieces that are the fields through which we will walk:

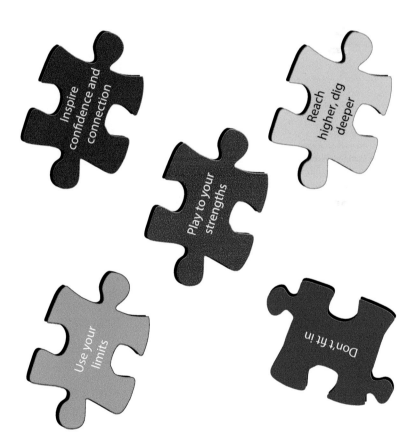

3

Reach higher, dig deeper

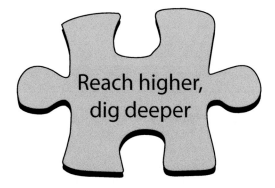

In this chapter, we will explore these questions:

- Why does inspiration matter and how might we use it?
- Isn't it sensible to cut our losses rather than fail?
- If we reach for the impossible, aren't we just mad?
- Where can we find the help to keep us going?
- What is the place of courage?
- Aren't good leaders also charismatic?

Have a care

As we said in the introduction to this section, as leaders we need to care about something that also matters to others, and also care about the people. We use the word 'care' in a number of senses. These include being concerned about, committed to and compassionate about. All of these forms of caring are important to other people and help them to connect to us. Caring is also vital to ourselves, because without it, we won't experience the motivation and energy that drive us to improve the situation or to help others.

What we care about may be diverse. For example, it may be poverty, inequality, injustice, isolation or being marginalised. Equally, it could be beauty, creativity, kindness and harmony. Whatever we care about, we can bring it into our work as leaders and use its energy to help the group succeed.

If we care about something strongly enough, we may find ourselves driven to lead the change and persuade others to the cause. As Irwin Corey said, 'If we don't change direction soon, we'll end up where we're going'.

If, as is commonly the case, we haven't chosen to lead but have had it 'thrust upon us', we can look for something within the enterprise that we genuinely find motivating.

Case example

The practice team was growing and the rota system was becoming unmanageable. Rona, a deputy manager, was given the task of revamping this and, initially, she thought the task would be tedious because her main interest was in people rather than IT and administration. However, she found a way of connecting with her main drive by reimagining the project as an opportunity to create a system that improved people's lives by giving adequate cover for workload and creating ways of accommodating time off. This gave her the motivation and energy to drive the project by convincing people of the need to change and provide support for the team to move forward. Despite the teething problems, the new system and her leadership were seen as really valuable and were appreciated.

If we don't try to find our motivation or don't succeed in doing so, although we may have a lead position and be a figure of authority and control, the fact that we don't care *enough* means that we are unlikely to become effective leaders.

Let's now move on to consider what inspires us and why this is also important.

Dream on

Leadership is one percent inspiration, ninety-nine percent perspiration.

Thomas Edison (paraphrased quotation)

Unlike with caring, leaders don't have to be inspired – but it helps. Inspiration has a connection with caring in that what inspires us, both shapes and reflects what we care about.

Can you bring to mind the feeling of being inspired? Maybe it came from someone you heard speak, or the feeling you had from being part of a group who were enthusiastic and passionate about a subject dear to you. For many, the feeling not only energises but cannot be contained. It drives us to *do* something with the energy it creates and, for a period, it makes us forget our fears and the blocks that stand in the way. This is why it matters.

As Edison pointed out, the road to significant improvement is long and tedious. To persist, we need energy, and inspiration may be the most potent if not the most prevalent, source. 'One percent inspiration' doesn't sound like much, but we could think of it as 'the difference that makes the difference'. It is like the one-degree gap between water and the steam that powered the Industrial Revolution.

Our reach should exceed our grasp.

Robert Browning

This is an inspiring message and it suggests to us as individuals and as a community that if we don't reach for the impossible, we won't go beyond what is currently possible. Put another way, if our reach is *within* our grasp, we may refine the present rather than reimagine the future.

Perhaps it also says something about the importance of our dreams. As we've suggested, leadership gives people the confidence that even when there are no 'solutions', we can reach for and attain something better than we currently have. Because our imagination is always a few steps ahead of what is currently possible, imagining something that is currently out of reach will stimulate the thinking that either gets us there, or at the least, somewhere nearer.

'Getting nearer' is in fact success, not failure, so imagine what the team could achieve if they understood and believed this. How might that transform their attitude to trying?

Later we will consider how we maintain our fortitude and resilience. Here, we suggest that to reach higher, we need to understand our passions, be open to being inspired to creating the circumstances to foster that. Here are two thoughts:

- Reasoning is the water that puts out the fire of inspiration. If we get too rational too early about an inspiring dream, we risk drowning its flame. We risk extinguishing the power that inspiration has to energise us to find a way of achieving our goal.
- Putting yourself in the company of inspiring people is great. Removing yourself from those who drain you, is also great.

So, as we've seen, inspiration is important; however, the everyday reality of leadership is that it can feel more like plodding than passion. Leadership doesn't just require us to initiate the process of change through inspiration, we also need to sustain it and this we do by being persistent.

Dig for victory

Many leaders fail because they did not realise how close they were to success when they gave up.

Thomas Edison

We want our teams to succeed because that's the point of leadership. Edison's quote suggests that the main difference between those who succeed for their teams and those who do not is not intelligence, creativity or indeed any particular skill. It is the ability to keep on going for five minutes longer than anyone else would have done, especially when others in our community are openly questioning our judgement in resolving to persevere.

Great leaders know this, too. Winston Churchill is said to have written 'KBO: Keep Buggering On' in the margin of his wartime notes to remind himself and others not to give up or give in.

Wartime Britain used the phrase 'digging for victory' and for leadership this means digging deeper by showing grit and determination. But what if these aren't a strong part of your character? Don't despair because, as the diagram below shows, we only have to look around us in life to find that help is always at hand.

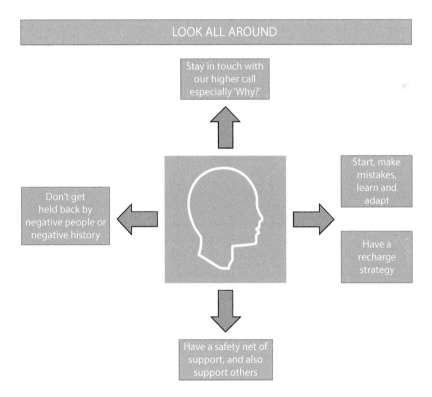

Let's briefly explore what we mean by 'looking around':

Look above: *Stay in touch with our higher call especially our 'Why?'.*

We shouldn't just do our job. Every day should have meaning and purpose or else life becomes a drudgery and if this sentiment means something important to us, it certainly will to our team. Make it happen, remind people of their 'Why'. We explore the 'Why' in Chapter 17.

Look ahead: *Start, make mistakes, learn and adapt. Recharge your batteries.*

We'll succeed, but it will take time. Persistence is about practical application and it's not compatible with rigidity because it's not about keeping on with the same plan but about exploring, adapting and evolving. We shouldn't assume that changing the plan will lead to a loss of face or be seen as a sign of failure. Quite the opposite; the less we deceive ourselves into being rigid, the fewer wrong roads we will persist in journeying along. Good leaders are also good *teachers* and the team can both be kept on board and can develop their capability further if these insights are shared and discussed.

Because feeling inspired makes us feel powerfully energised and activated, we should notice when, where and how this occurs and then build those circumstances into our lives.

More practically, a plan, with time put aside in our diaries to recharge our batteries routinely rather than by chance, will keep us physically and emotionally well and will maintain momentum.

Case example

Roger found he became periodically run down, which not only affected his ability to cope well with the work but also to maintain his optimism. He recognised that having time with his friends, taking short breaks or walking in the country helped him to feel happy and positive. So, he started colour-coding his diary using the colour yellow for his 'treats' and was quickly able to eyeball where these were in the months ahead. This kept his spirits up because he could see when the treats were coming. He could also plan ahead and make sure that the fun happened frequently enough to stop him getting rundown inadvertently.

Look below: *Have a safety net of support, and also support others.*

We all need a net of people: for mutual stimulation, to share resources and to support us especially when we feel we are falling. Talking to trusted friends also helps by putting our doubts into perspective. Also, keeping a file of positive feedback that we have had from patients, colleagues and others and using this to lift our mood at moments when we feel dispirited, can remind us that we are valued and can help us to maintain our confidence. This is not a sign of weakness or immaturity but simply of being human, because most of us need positive strokes, to some degree, to get through each day.

And of course, as others help us, we help them. We are part of other people's nets and good leaders always support others, including other leaders.

Don't look back: *Don't get held back by negative people or negative history.*

When we think about negative people in our lives, it is worth reminding ourselves that negative feedback, offered constructively, isn't negative. People who stop us going off the rails are not holding us back but are keeping us moving forward. It's hard sometimes to appreciate that, after all, no one likes criticism.

However, there are those who will drain us or seek to bring us down; ultimately, we may feel that they are not people we can trust. They may be negative because of their own problems and issues, but nevertheless there are times when it's okay to cut ourselves loose.

There are many stories of failure, including ones that we keep alive because they happened to ourselves. Although it's hard, we do have a choice. If we are committed to learn from experience rather than, for example, evoking self-pity, then history need not repeat itself.

Being courageous

Leadership involves moving out of our comfort zone and deliberately feeling uncomfortable, not because we are masochistic but because stretching ourselves allows us to learn, grow and forge a better path. That's an important outcome and makes the pain (in retrospect) seem worthwhile. If the move from our comfort zone is accompanied by significant *risk* then we don't just need energy to do it, we also need courage. Reaching higher and digging deeper are both actions that call for courage, so maybe we should ask ourselves whether, if we rarely feel uncomfortable or need to use our courage, we are actually engaging in leadership at all.

Courage isn't just for those who are extraordinary; it's an everyday activity conducted by everyday people. It's widespread and often low-profile. For example, people show courage when they:

- Try to be their real selves
- Take risks
- Seek out feedback
- Step aside and let others shine
- Influence those with power
- Keep trying
- Show their vulnerability

Looking back, which of these have you done and did you have to be courageous in doing so? Doing such things and recognising that it can lead to really positive outcomes helps us to be courageous, reach higher and be brave in riskier situations.

Our courage is there to help us achieve something important, but it doesn't have to be used alone; it's simply one of a number of tools. We can be more effective still if we add skills and intelligence to our ability to be bold. For example, by building a stock of goodwill so that people are more likely to support us, by looking for an opportune moment such as when those with power are more approachable, or by choosing the right battle rather than being indiscriminate.

Likewise, why use more courage than we have to? For instance, we can help ourselves in risky situations by preparing as best we can, so that the *need* for courage is minimised. Or we can consider whether resorting to courage is actually appropriate. Inappropriate courage can make us foolhardy and take risks in situations where we needn't.

To give an example, inappropriate courage can make us rely on our ability to 'wing it' rather than put the effort into preparing properly, say for a presentation or a coaching session. People notice when this happens because inadequate preparation often has adverse consequences. As a result, instead of creating confidence in people through our actions, we can end up undermining confidence through our unnecessary risk-taking.

Whatever the outcome of the struggle in which we've had to use courage, after the event we should be civil and kind to those involved. Today's adversaries could be tomorrow's allies and vice versa, so it's wise to show that we value our long-term relationships and that these are more important to us than the shorter-term conflicts.

Case example

Aileen, a junior receptionist, had been working on a new system of text messaging to alert patients of abnormal test results and to allow them to repeat these without having to make a surgery appointment. The practice manager, Kevin, couldn't implement the recommendations in the way that she had recommended and this upset her greatly. She was courageous in challenging him and he shared with her that there were other issues that were standing in the way, which he explained. Rather than falling out, Aileen told Kevin that she understood his difficult position and was ready to take the project forward when the time was right.

Helping people to make better choices: inspiration, not charisma

Leadership isn't just how we see ourselves. It is as much a quality that others attribute to us, which means that, in a real sense, leadership is bestowed on us by the choices that others make.

We can influence such choices by 'reaching higher and digging deeper'. Through this we can become people who inspire others rather than merely entertain or 'wow' them through attempting to be charismatic. Despite society's cult of personality, leadership is not so much about the persona of the leader (the ego) but the environment or relationship between leader and team (the eco). Leaders who inspire are not so much concerned with cultivating their celebrity as with showing the daily commitment that builds long-term relationships and liberates the potential of others.

Charisma is highly effective but only in the short-term, as although it energises people, it shortcuts the relationship that needs to develop between leader and team for them to work well together. In this sense, charisma resembles infatuation.

But rather than disparage charisma, we can learn from it. Thus, whilst avoiding the temptation to impress people, we can take a leaf out of charisma's book in learning to communicate and connect more powerfully. For example, we can simplify and give hope in difficult situations. We can be clear about our collective vision, be direct about how we are getting there and upbeat and courageous in communicating our confidence of success. If these behaviours are underpinned by our concern and commitment for our team, we can help them to build trust and avoid taking refuge in false hopes, based on the false impressions that facades like charisma create.

Over the stile

Reaching higher to what inspires and drives us and digging deeper by being committed to helping and supporting people, provide a solid basis for getting the job done. We may excite or interest people to make a difference, but how do we keep them on board when success is not easily or quickly achieved?

In the next chapter we explore how our attitudes and behaviour, even more than our skills, are central to maintaining the trust and confidence of our colleagues. We may not possess these to the optimal degree, we may never do so, but we will discuss their importance so that we feel encouraged, and able, to improve. Let's move on.

4

Inspire confidence and connection

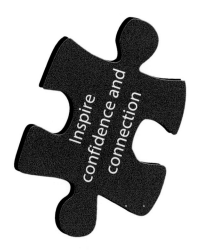

In this chapter, we will explore these questions:

- Why are trust and confidence needed?
- How might people develop trust in us?
- Isn't 'putting on a good front' necessary for people to have confidence in us?
- How could we foster our integrity?
- How can people have confidence in our ability as leaders?
- How can we nurture our self-confidence?
- What can we do, and stop doing, to connect better with people?
- Aren't errors, failures and vulnerabilities bad in leaders?
- How can we balance our ego and appreciate others better?

Why do we need confidence and connection?

Perhaps this is the most important jigsaw piece of all, so let's consider why.

Leaders and teams need to have confidence in each other and to want to connect with each other. That way, the practice moves forward. But what are the factors that foster confidence and connection? We will discuss these mainly from the viewpoint of leaders, although the notions are applicable to everyone in the team.

Because the problems we face in primary care are complex with no guaranteed solutions, people need to trust each other in order to experiment with routes forward. Trust is needed in order to live with uncertainty and risk, and people tend to place their trust in other *people*, for example colleagues in their leaders, more than in *processes*. For the purposes of this discussion, we suggest that people broadly base their trust and confidence on someone's integrity and ability; good leaders need to have both.

We will look first at integrity and ability, and later move on to consider why *connection* is important and how we can nurture people's willingness to collaborate with us.

Integrity

Integrity is important for everyone, not just for clinicians and professionals. It means trying to live by a strong moral and ethical code, for example in not telling lies, not breaking confidences, not knowingly doing harm, trying to do good and being committed to fairness and justice.

Integrity means being open about our values and trying to live by what we claim is important. In addition, it means being *honest*, especially about those times when we fall short, which being human we will often do.

At a deeper level still, integrity relates to the degree to which we try and become whole, integrated people by:

- Being open to discover more about who and what we are,
- Being ourselves and not knowingly trying to deceive ourselves or others,
- Trying to 'integrate' the way we live with what we claim to believe,
- Accepting ourselves, warts and all.

Potential followers look closely for this and nothing undermines the trust that people have in us more than a perceived lack of integrity, for example being 'two-faced'. This is not surprising, after all how can others believe in (let alone follow) someone who isn't what they claim to be?

Integrity in all its manifestations is therefore the foundation of a leader's reputation and once lost, it can be almost impossible to regain. Therefore, let's explore how we can nurture our integrity and become people who are more worthy of the trust of others and of our own self-belief.

As we do this, let's remind ourselves not to be too harsh with ourselves or, indeed, too forgiving.

Being open to discover more about who and what we are

Being open helps us to understand ourselves better and puts us in a position to be more honest about ourselves, which is a key component of integrity. Being open breeds trust and we can therefore become more effective both as individuals and as a team when we are more open with each other. It takes courage to engage in this process, disclose sensitive things about ourselves and be willing to hear the perceptions that others have of us. As with much else that we discuss in this chapter, our personal attempts to improve act as an example that encourages others in the team to consider their own behaviour and also challenge their willingness to improve.

Based on Johari's window (1), there are three really useful ways of getting a better understanding of who we are and of helping others see that we are not trying to hide or to protect ourselves. The point being that the more we learn about ourselves, the more effectively we can use our attributes and tailor our influence to help others:

1   We can get *feedback* about what people think of us, so we are less *blinkered*. Giving feedback is a difficult task and can be helped if the people we ask are clear about the purpose and the area of our behaviour that they are being asked to comment upon. Rather than starting by identifying a person, we can define what we need to receive feedback about, for example our ability to delegate or to chair a meeting, then identify colleagues who have witnessed enough of this to legitimately comment.

2   Of those available, we can then invite someone who will give feedback in a balanced and constructive way and will not use the opportunity for their own ends or to undermine us. In addition, seeking feedback from people such as friends and mentors who know us well, care about us and can be honest, helps us to develop and keep on track. Only from people whom we trust the most can we ask one of the most revealing questions about ourselves: 'What is it like to be on the receiving end of me?'

3   Being selective in this way about receiving feedback, so as to avoid unnecessary harm, is not cowardly but intelligent and legitimate.

4   We can *open up* about ourselves, maybe by sharing something about ourselves that is personal, even vulnerable, so that we put up less of a

façade. This can be done in formal settings, for example in meetings, but it is much easier and less risky to do in social situations, hence the importance of mixing with colleagues socially so that we can get to know and trust each other.

5 As leaders, because we recognise the importance of this, we may need to prioritise and plan these trust-building social interactions, rather than hope that they happen. This becomes particularly important when new groups form, as we discuss in Chapter 13.

6 Sometimes there are things we don't know about ourselves and that others haven't noticed or can't know. Although they don't appeal to everyone, there are *tools*, such as personality or competence assessments, that can explore this area so that we have less of a *blind spot*.

The more open we are about ourselves, the more honest we are seen to be and the less our ignorance about ourselves is mistaken for knowing deception.

In addition to getting feedback from others, people use 360 feedback, which includes *self*-assessment. It is natural for people to under- or overestimate themselves, but with time, experience and more exposure to the views of others, we can learn to be more accurate and balanced with our self-assessment.

Self-awareness is an essential tool for developing the insight that helps us to improve. As leaders, if we can be seen to be open-minded enough to learn, others can maintain their confidence in us because however worrying the situation and at times our behaviour, they can see we have the ability to learn and improve.

Clarifying who and what we are at our core is difficult because we don't really notice when we are just being ourselves. However, we could use our self-awareness to notice when we are *not* being ourselves and appreciate how that compromises our connection with others. By doing less of this and thereby being less inauthentic, we reciprocally become more ourselves.

Case example

John often found, maybe out of nervousness or insecurity, that he overpraised people, sometimes giving them credit where it wasn't due or saying something positive about them when actually, he was ducking a difficult conversation. Although he thought he was being kind, he recognised that this was harming him because actually, he wasn't being honest. This began to affect his self-respect but he turned this round by noticing when he was about to say something he didn't

(Continued)

mean and then stopping himself from doing so. His change in behaviour was noticed by others and he was seen as being more sincere and honest, rather than 'unkind' and this helped him become more effective. It wasn't until he changed his behaviour that John appreciated that some people had previously viewed him as being insincere and dishonest. This was a shock to him as he didn't imagine people would notice, but it made him resolve to be more open in the future.

Self-awareness doesn't just show us what we *are*, but by pointing up the areas in which we are being inauthentic, it shows us what we are *not*.

Getting to discover our real selves also means learning about ourselves beyond the workplace. This is because being a *person* is always bigger than being a leader, manager, or any other *work* role. It's also bigger than any *life* role such as parent, child, partner and so on, although some of the most important parts of our identity come from these. Whatever its importance, no role should define us. Because our identity is deeper than this, we need to think outside the constraints of our roles and reconsider ourselves, for example by clarifying what drives us when we are freer of the expectations that we, and others, place upon us.

In order to learn more about themselves, some people seek to be vulnerable, which is a brave thing to do, by putting themselves in situations outside the work context where their rank, qualifications, achievements and influence are not known. This could include clubs, societies and volunteering activities.

By learning to be helpful through using our social skills, rather than relying on our status or CV to do the heavy lifting for us, we can gain a less filtered perspective on our nature and abilities. Importantly, stripping ourselves of rank also helps us to appreciate the qualities of others and experience the humility that gives us a more balanced perspective on our own place in society.

All of these methods of discovery require time to reflect so that we can integrate what we learn and acquire a deeper understanding. It's important to remember that reflection is stimulated as much through talking with others as through having quiet time to think things through on our own. *Everyone* is capable of reflecting, it's just that we find different ways of doing this that suit our preferences. In addition, if we can practise pausing to reflect *in* the moment rather than just back *on* the moment, we can become more effective by being wise in the event, rather than just wise *after* the event.

Being ourselves and not knowingly deceiving ourselves or others

> To thine own self be true.
>
> **Polonius in Shakespeare's *Hamlet***

There are two components here that impact upon our integrity. First, there is the absolute importance of not trying to deceive people by claiming to be what we know we are not. This behaviour damages trust, even if it is well-intentioned.

The second is discovering and being our true selves, which is sometimes referred to as being genuine or authentic. Behaving in this way makes us a more 'whole' person, someone who is prepared to respect and accept themselves and stop chasing an illusion or be seduced or obligated by what others would like us to be. Such a person is also more likely to value and nurture the authenticity of others.

Let's suggest a caveat that being true to ourselves also has to be socially acceptable, although philosophers would debate that point vigorously of course. For example, evil and cruelty might be genuinely dominant aspects of a person's character, but we recognise that each society has behaviours that it cannot condone. In our leadership context, being genuine is about trying to connect with our deeper selves, living within society's code but not being defined by it.

As is said, if you fake it, you won't make it. However, the tendency to put up a façade and pretend to be what we are not is everywhere in society and is not easy to guard against. For instance, look at how people portray themselves on social media, or the way we readily accept the false image that flattery creates. Our human insecurity makes it natural to believe in high praise but this makes it harder to appreciate and value our true selves. If we are misled about ourselves, we will mis-*lead* others.

Faking it is particularly damaging where it relates to our deeper features, such as our values, attitudes, beliefs and ability. Therefore, when we espouse certain ideals and then don't live up to them, or pretend to be more gifted, clever, expert or connected then we are, we can quickly lose trust when we are found out.

Sometimes pretence can come from a good place. It's quite understandable to think, as leaders, that it's necessary to put on a front for the sake of our colleagues. For instance, to pretend to have confidence in people or projects in order to instil confidence in others.

However well-meaning, in a community that is based on trust, it isn't appropriate or we could argue ultimately effective, to try and fool people.

We 'leak' all the time through non-verbal language, unguarded comments, inconsistent behaviour and so on, so being found out isn't just possible, it's inevitable. It's really a matter of when, not if. Here's an example:

Case example

Simon, the senior partner, has fallen out with Kate, his practice manager, over a financial issue. There have been no public arguments, but the tension between them is unsettling the staff. When Simon is asked if everything is all right, he thinks he's reassuring them by saying, 'I don't know what you are talking about, everything's fine', but they notice that he avoids eye contact and looks nervous. Far from feeling reassured, they start to lose confidence in him and the senior team.

Sometimes the façade comes not from an intention to deceive people but from the anxiety or even fear that we have to present ourselves as leaders in a way that is acceptable to others, such as by appearing tough, courageous or entertaining.

For instance, one aspect of being genuine is public speaking. Most leaders are anxious about speaking to large groups, but those that do it well don't worry about their image or being entertaining but try to connect with the audience from their deeper selves, especially from their values and beliefs.

So, if pretence is to be avoided, how can we discover our real selves? Here are some questions that encourage us to become more aware of our identity:

- What have you hidden or denied? In other words, what have you hidden that you would prefer others not to know and what have you heard about yourself that you have pretended to yourself has no basis?

- Take one aspect of the 'real' you that you find uncomfortable. How could you reflect that aspect, with honesty, in the way you live?

- Can you give an example of when you are aware you are *not* being true to yourself? For instance, when you say what you don't mean or deliberately hide or mislead, perhaps with good intentions but then again, perhaps not.

- How do you feel about that? And has anyone noticed?

- What about when you go along with other people's designs on you? Why do you do that? For example, you may feel you owe it to them or that you need to comply in order to advance your career.

- How could you share your vulnerability (which we all have) and how might this help you to be more genuine?

As we learn from this, we will be more ourselves and less how we would like to be seen, and that is a good thing. The need for façade will become less because being ourselves and being vulnerable will nurture connections and help people understand us better. It will also model to others that being genuine, although difficult, is not only possible but important.

Accepting ourselves, warts and all

> Because true belonging only happens when we present our authentic, imperfect selves to the world; our sense of belonging can never be greater than our level of self-acceptance.
>
> **Brené Brown**

If we don't truly accept ourselves, it's harder for others to do so. We are often our own worst critic, but accepting ourselves, including our darker recesses and our inner struggles, can help us to grow. For example, through accepting such feelings as self-importance or envy, rather than pretending they don't exist, we can learn not to feed them more than they demand. Thereby, they have a less damaging effect on ourselves and others and ultimately, their demands may fade.

Accepting ourselves is a manifestation of honesty and therefore of integrity. Through it, we are calmer and more stable because we are not blown about by the winds of what other people think of us or by the frustration that we feel about ourselves. Acceptance may come through exhaustion but it may equally come through wisdom, which guides and stabilises without controlling.

Leaders who can accept themselves and be open about their weaknesses whilst striving to be better, are remarkable. They show through their example that it's not only okay but also important to be human and that it's our vulnerability as well as our strengths that make us uniquely valuable to each other.

At a broader level, good leadership helps us to accept *who* we are, whilst not necessarily accepting *how* we are. Ultimately, rather than feeling resigned to accept ourselves, we may feel thankful to have developed into what we have become.

Confidence in ability

We said earlier that trust and confidence are not only based on our integrity but also on our ability, which for us means the ability to lead successfully through having the necessary knowledge, skills, attitudes and behaviours. Competence, especially in professionals, is often assumed to be present unless proven otherwise. However, even though our competence as leaders may not be questioned, that doesn't mean it isn't noticed.

Competence affects trust in a different way to integrity. Someone who is persistently incompetent can't be trusted to deliver, not because they are a 'bad person' but because they don't have the tools to do so. We may not think that this could apply to us, but *competence* in performing well decays much more quickly than our *confidence* or belief that our performance is up to the mark. Competence needs to be checked rather than assumed and when needed, restored through education and training. Therefore, people who underperform, which is all of us at some point, can continue to be trusted if they are seen to keep their performance under review and to attend to deficiencies.

If gauging our performance helps people to maintain their confidence in us, how might we assist that process? In a nutshell, our leadership performance is a combination of how we handle two major areas: people and task. Let's consider them both.

Our behaviour and the way others are with us, give a good indication of our interpersonal skills and our performance with *people*. These skills include our ability to develop relationships, communicate well and use self-awareness and self-control, particularly of our emotions. We don't have to draw people's attention to how we perform in this area, as this may be misinterpreted and is unnecessary as our 'people ability' is quickly noticed and reflected in our reputation.

Our *task* ability is ultimately gauged through our ability to deliver, which requires skills beyond managing people, such as problem-solving, planning and organising. We can help others to form their opinion by making sure that progress with tasks is not only occurring but also is seen to be occurring.

People and task abilities are complementary and good performance in one can reduce the burden on the other. For example, when people can see from data on wall charts that the new way of care navigating is reducing the wait for face-to-face appointments, they will depend less on 'people-skills' such as explanation and persuasion to feel confident of progress and engaged with change.

As well as competence, *consistency* of behaviour is also important because it helps people to feel more confident in situations that are uncertain or where the outcomes are not yet clear. It would be very hard if the team not only had to cope with uncertain situations but were being led by leaders who were themselves unpredictable. We read the news. We only have to look at the political or financial worlds to see how devastating unpredictability can be in preventing people from planning or having confidence in their futures. Unpredictable leaders have unhappy and incapable teams. That part is predictable.

Being consistent partly means making the same decision in the same circumstances, which is really important with some issues such as calling those people to account who break the rules, don't meet agreed commitments and so on. Team members look very closely at how we manage such situations and appropriately consistent behaviour is fundamental to reassuring people of our fairness.

However, sometimes our actions are *different* in the same circumstances because we have changed as a result of learning. If we don't want our team to lose confidence in us because they think we are being inconsistent, we would be wise to anticipate this, acknowledge that we are doing things differently and explain why our judgement or behaviour has changed. In this way we can also model *adaptability*, a key skill for successful teams.

Confidence begins at home: a note on self-confidence

Through attending to our deeper features of integrity and ability, other people come to develop trust and confidence in us. In addition, our own self-confidence becomes well-founded and robust.

However, this process is long and requires great personal commitment so it is not surprising that many leaders, particularly early on in their leadership career, lack confidence in themselves especially when they step up to new challenges. One manifestation of this is the so-called impostor syndrome. This is not a bad thing, because it tempers arrogance and encourages humility, as a result of which we connect better with others.

However, our confidence needs to be 'good enough' not to be an impediment and here are some ways of encouraging that:

- Talking to others and discovering that a lack of self-confidence is ubiquitous. This is reassuring and helps put our own feelings into perspective.
- We may not feel up to the role of leadership even when others encourage us, particularly when we first consider becoming 'visible' as leaders. However, we are more experienced than we realise. Because leadership is about helping others to make a difference, we

can learn to appreciate that there have been situations and communities in which we have already done that. These are likely to be many and may include friendship, sport, church or social groups. Because our leadership experience is broader, longer and more effective than we thought, we have the evidence to believe in ourselves more strongly than we imagined.

- The leadership skills that we learn in one context can be transferred and built upon in another, thereby boosting our self-efficacy and self-belief. For clinicians, the consultation is one important example of this and is discussed in Chapter 5.

- Having a go is all-important. Rather than just dwelling on the challenges, if we can apply our leadership skills and later debrief on the experience, we can quickly improve our performance and confidence. Ideally, we should seek a coach or mentor who can counsel and debrief, and this person will often be a leader of greater experience. In fact, it is a vital part of our own leadership role that in due course we help other leaders in this way.

- Self-confidence needs continual maintenance. If we take notice of what boosts our confidence, especially those things we do that are valuable to others, we can bring these more frequently into our lives. Significant achievements are fine, but it is often the smaller less noticeable personal acts, like helping individuals, that keep us buoyant.

Connection

Being worthy of the trust and confidence of our colleagues may mean that we have earned their respect, but it does not mean that we have gained their desire to willingly connect with us and collaborate to improve. Let us now look at a number of ways in which we can improve relationships and foster the desire to connect.

Power and vulnerability: reducing the gap

In order to relate better, we must first avoid disconnecting.

Leadership is intrinsically separating and then alienating, as both leaders and their teams come to view each other differently because of their roles. Leadership can, if misapplied, encourage leaders to embrace their strengths and spurn their weaknesses. Both actions are dangerous because the combination of high power and low vulnerability increases the gap between leaders and the rest of the team and is toxic to collaboration.

Status, rank and power accentuate strength and a sense of superiority, which separate us and eventually diminish the desire to connect with our colleagues. How important is our status to us? To explore this, we might consider how we feel when people don't know our rank. We might also reflect on whether we signal our status socially, for example by using our titles when shopping or making reservations.

One of the problems with higher status is that almost universally, people find it hard to 'speak up to power'. Some leaders may see this barrier as a benefit of course, but the barrier means that we can not only become disconnected, but also misled. Even if we don't seek to parade our power, status can make others less honest and open with us, for example about less helpful aspects of our influence or the realities of what's going wrong or how people are feeling in the workplace.

If taking care over status can reduce the gap, then so can sharing our vulnerability. We are all vulnerable and being able to share that is not weakness, but a sign that we don't see ourselves as being different but as being like everyone else. Importantly, being vulnerable gives people a way of connecting, through compassion, with those who although more powerful, are equally human.

We can become better leaders by being honest about our fears, weaknesses and mistakes and also at times by showing our wounds. Through this process, we may develop greater compassion for ourselves as well as others and come to appreciate that strength doesn't come from believing that we can avoid falling down, but in knowing that we will always try to get up.

Case example

Izzy was a forceful deputy manager but found that although the team achieved results, she often alienated people. This was fed back to her in appraisal and she turned things around by saying to her team, 'Look, I've messed up but I'm really going to try and change. It won't be easy for me as I'm not the easiest to get on with. However, I will try to get better so please help me and bear with me when I get it wrong'. Izzy's openness, especially about her vulnerability, changed attitudes to her overnight.

Being fair to people

Any behaviour that threatens our integrity, like unfairness, is likely to diminish the desire that people have to connect and relate to us. However, in this section, the focus is not so much on the unethical behaviour of being unfair or discriminatory as on how to take active steps to recognise our biases, *avoid* unfairness and treat people well.

Biases are our inclinations for or against people, ideas, behaviours and so on. They are often unconscious, and therefore may be unintentional, and we all have them. Contrary to what we might think, biases are natural and many are useful. Like assumptions, they are shortcuts that help us to quickly assess people and situations so that we can take action. We need them because the brain receives millions of bits of information per second of which our conscious minds can only deal with about 50. As a result, without mental shortcuts we would quickly be paralysed by information overload. Therefore, we shouldn't be too hard on ourselves because bias isn't inherently bad, unnatural or avoidable. It is as much about our biology as our ethics.

As we can see, bias is partly the result of necessity. Through becoming conscious of where we are biased and where we make assumptions, we can respect and retain the ones that are useful and attend to those that we discover are damaging.

Bias can be damaging because it narrows the options that we allow ourselves, and thereby becomes excluding. For example, if we are unhelpfully biased about *information*, this might narrow our thinking and the decisions we are prepared to contemplate. With *groups of people*, bias might narrow the range of people that we choose to work with, which also means that by excluding some, we favour others. 'Affinity bias' which is widespread and refers to the tendency to prefer people who are like us, is a common example of this. With *individuals*, unhelpful bias might narrow our perception of their talents and how we might make best use of them. Bias blinkers our way of seeing people and can result in favour being shown to some at the expense of fewer opportunities and support being offered to others. Unsurprisingly, this is likely to be interpreted as unfairness.

Prejudice has more significant implications because it is a conscious preconceived opinion, literally a pre-judgement that may not be based on knowledge, reason or experience. It matters because it can lead to discrimination. We could ask ourselves: Who are the people or 'types' that I instinctively dislike, or like? When I come across them, what if anything can I do to avoid being unfair?

Unfairness and discrimination seriously undermine the confidence and trust that people have in us and to raise our awareness so we can then minimise them, we could:

- **Become aware of our blind spots.** Through feedback, we can assess whether our unconscious biases are becoming problematic. Such feedback is hard to ask for and hard to give, even by people more powerful than ourselves. However, if we create a safe space for people, they can be encouraged to do so without damaging repercussions. Additionally, if we listen out, we can hear people comment on our traits informally, particularly in social situations. For example, we can take notice of how people tease us. Sometimes they are pointing out something about ourselves that would be difficult or dangerous to say formally.

Another way of seeing if unconscious bias is damaging is through looking at an event where a problem has occurred and tracking back to identify the unhelpful assumptions and biases that may have contributed to it.

- **Become aware of biases,** if it suits the ways we like to learn, through online tests such as 'Project Implicit' run though Harvard University (2). This is very interesting and probes how we instinctively react to such things as gender, race, disability, religion, weight, age, etc. The responses are important because they demonstrate that bias is ubiquitous and the results can be an eye-opener in showing how instinctively and unconsciously, we judge each other.

If we are able to share our self-awareness more openly, we may also find that preferences that we recognise in ourselves can lead us to judge others in ways we may not be so conscious of. For instance, by preferring:

- Compassion over being tough on people, we may consider those who do the latter as being **cruel**
- Being balanced over being flattering we may consider those who do the latter as being **deceitful**
- Being thoughtful over being amusing we may consider those who are the latter as being **trivial**

Some biases have a damaging effect on leadership because they incline us to modify our goals. For example, 'safety' bias encourages us to choose the safer option and often this is driven by fear of what we might lose. Knowing this allows us to both correct for the tendency and to be more effective in persuading other people of the need for change. We can do the latter by recognising the safety bias in others and taking time to explore what they might be fearful of losing such as money, status, influence or importance in a group. In addition, we can explain the need for change not only in terms of what we might gain if we do, but what we might lose if we don't.

In addition, people are subject to 'distance' bias, where distance refers to both time and place. For example, we are more likely to favour short-termism, i.e., a gain in the short term rather than something more substantial in the longer term. The proverb 'a bird in the hand is worth two in the bush' reflects this tendency. Also, we favour communities, services, people, etc., that are closer geographically rather than those that are further away.

- **Learn not to act from assumptions.** For example, we all use stereotypes, which are premature judgements about an individual made on the basis of the category that we quickly decide they fall into. Sometimes these are helpful in allowing us to respond well to someone before we get to know them but often, they shortcut our need to relate and thereby make us respond inappropriately and connect badly.

For example, we might think 'Oh, he had a private education, so he's going to be arrogant and feel entitled'. Conversely, we might think the opposite. Instead, we can use *self-awareness* to recognise when we are about to jump to a conclusion and then use *self-discipline* to hit the pause button and find out more about the person and situation first.

Rather than think of stereotypes as being 'wrong', it can be more helpful to think of them as being incomplete. They *may* contain some truth, but not enough to be relied upon. We can use them as a starting point if we have no other information, but supplement them by getting other perspectives to form a more complete picture. As with all forms of assumption, the more information we have, the less we have to rely upon potentially toxic shortcuts.

Another assumption is our tendency for an impression created in one area to influence opinion in another area. A good example of this is the halo and horn effect. In the former, we might inappropriately assume that if someone is good in one area, they will be good in another unrelated area and this might lead us to offer opportunities that are inappropriate. With the horn effect, the opposite applies.

- *Become aware of our triggers*, especially those things that prompt us to be too negative or too positive. One insight that can help to raise our awareness is that we can be particularly negative about those characteristics in others that we struggle to accept in ourselves. If you imagine this doesn't apply to you, think about what you find most irritating in those closest to you, like your parents or siblings. Generally speaking, if we are triggered by other people, this may be saying more about us than about them.
- *Challenge our attitudes.* We can meet, socialise and work with a broader range of people, learn to value them and thereby come to appreciate more of humanity as 'us', not 'them'. This opens our hearts and minds to the need to create opportunities to use a broader range of people and talent in our leadership work.

How does this apply to leadership in real life? Here are a couple of examples of leaders, their personal biases and the influence these have:

OUR NEGATIVE BIAS	WHAT OUR COLLEAGUE MIGHT FEEL
We show prejudice against women, and have referred to senior colleagues as 'silly schoolgirls'.	I'm shocked at what I hear. He does it rarely and only with other men, but when he talks about equality and respect, I don't believe him because I've heard for myself what he's really like.
Young people are one of our triggers. We get irritated by them, their attitudes and behaviours. We say they don't show the commitment that we did when we were young, they're always on their phones and they can't focus on anything for more than five minutes.	It's good that the leader tells it like it is. It's about time someone put these shirkers in their place.

You know how it is; we often imagine that people don't notice our negative bias. Furthermore, we might imagine that if colleagues *do* notice, then they will not think too badly of us; after all it just shows we're human doesn't it? We would be wrong on both counts and that's even before social media magnifies our behaviour out of all proportion. The hard fact is that as leaders we are expected to set the tone and to be role-models for the values of our organisation.

In the first example, the leader's behaviour is devastating to the female community and to those who can't abide sexism or patronising behaviour. Small comments, said in semi-private can undermine relationships that have taken years to build.

In the second example, the leader's behaviour has been approved of. This is just as bad, because the effect of the leader's prejudice is to legitimise and therefore reinforce the prejudice of others, which undermines trust even more widely though the team.

Being more open and not blocking the community's progress

Moving forward requires the community and therefore each individual, to flow. Otto Scharmer (3) characterised this in terms of encouraging each of us to open up and develop a mind that is open to ideas and possibilities, a heart that cares about and encourages others and a will that is open to changes happening.

The more open we become in these three dimensions, the stronger the connection that people have with us and with each other and the stronger the 'flow' of collaborative improvement. Opening up helps everyone to share and become better informed, which reduces our reliance on the shortcuts of assumptions and unhelpful bias. Put another way, opening up makes us place fewer conditions on what we are prepared to consider or who we are prepared to work with, because the more we know, the less we fear.

If only such openness was our default tendency, but generally it is not. For a host of reasons including fear, mean-spiritedness and ignorance, we can block each dimension. In the following section, we consider each of these more closely and how some blocks might be overcome.

Open mind

To be open-minded means valuing the information, ideas and interpretations that are in the literature or that people bring to the community. People are the repositories of diverse ideas which between them can help us solve problems and move forward. Being open-minded stops us from closing others down or closing ourselves off to thoughts that might help us to adapt as a community.

Of course, being closed-minded is not always a bad thing. Every behaviour has its place and closed minds can stop us from being distracted, it helps us to stick to our guns and even help us be more courageous when we are fearful or facing pressure. However, people do not connect well if they think mindsets are *persistently* closed as being so makes us more rigid, dogmatic and less likely to include people or consider other ways of dealing with a problem.

There are blocks to an open mind that we can help ourselves to overcome. Premature judgement can get in the way. We need to learn to pause, suspend judgement and give ourselves a chance to be more open-minded and therefore receptive to the information around us.

Opening our minds means opening our eyes to what is around us and opening our eyes can also mean opening them to the eyes of others:

Case example

Amit, one of the GP trainers, brought in a 'Fresh pair of eyes' (FPE) system for new trainees. In the first month, they had to find out about the practice, its people, culture and systems and then report to a team meeting. In the meeting, they identified two things they thought were great and could be adopted by other practices and one thing that they had reservations about or could be done better, based on what they had seen in other practices and teams. The exercise was a great success. Trainees assimilated far quicker into the practice, their recommendations were discussed and usually actioned and the trainees were given opportunities to make changes. Just at a time when, as newbies, they could have felt like a spare part, the trainees felt really valued and the scheme was quickly extended to include all new members of the team.

Scientists have a phrase 'let the data decide'. This tells us firstly that having information is important and reminds us of the absolute importance of being receptive to information by being alert and noticing things around us.

Secondly, it tells us that we should not prematurely put our spin on what we notice, but pause in order to become better informed. Seeking information is about being sufficiently interested to ask, and then to listen to people. This sounds straightforward but in reality, we often silence other people, particularly through our non-verbal communication. To listen, we have to stop closing people down and provide safety and encouragement for them to open up and share thoughts.

Although it happens, we should not feel disheartened or surprised that it takes time to let go of our old self. That resistance becomes less the more we recognise the blocks, keep pushing away at them and appreciate how we grow as a result. As leaders, we can help ourselves and others to become more open-minded. Here are a few ways:

- Be comfortable with being vulnerable and not 'knowing' and use this to be open to new information. Don't beat ourselves up for not having the 'right answers' but look for ideas elsewhere. Good leaders will model this by encouraging people to network, explore what is being done elsewhere, look at the research, etc., and report back.

- Admit when things aren't going as hoped. Don't make the data fit the hypothesis or the expectations. Every new approach is an experiment, not a solution, and remembering this can help us to legitimately rebrand 'failure' as 'learning'. If we do this, it can both encourage honesty and maintain morale.

- Encourage people to read and learn more widely than the health service. Although it's huge, the health service is still a silo with its own groupthink which constrains our insight and narrows our vision, especially about opportunities and ways of problem-solving.

- Ask ourselves, as evidence of the presence of an open-minded culture: Do people feel able to speak freely to me and to each other? How often do I hear opinions that are different from the majority? Do I promote this by showing appreciation of different ways of thinking and interacting?

Many of these approaches stem from having the courage to admit to not knowing it all. It's amazing how much stronger we all become when we are able to say 'I don't know, please help' or 'We got it wrong, what could we try next?' These simple words transform a culture by showing that ignorance can be the greatest teacher of all and is the key to new possibilities.

We might believe that the accusation of not being open-minded enough doesn't apply to us personally, but is that likely? Let's think for a moment about 'confirmation bias', which like most people, leaders are subject to. What this means is that we naturally listen out for and take more notice of information that confirms what we already believe. It's a powerful bias and inhibits us from being as open-minded as we need to be. It's a bit like 'groupthink', which is the practice of denying our different opinions and claiming to think the same, perhaps because out of a desire for harmony or the understandable wish to avoid conflict.

Open heart

At the level of the heart, being open means feeling sufficiently connected to people to trust and care about them. Caring matters because without it, we are less likely to want to persist with the hard graft of progress. It's a nice idea, but what are some of the blocks to that?

If you look, cynicism and blame are widespread and what these do is to make us mistrust other people and care more about our self-interest. To assist ourselves, we can learn to recognise our impulse to be cynical and to blame, especially when others are doing so, and stop ourselves from going down that path.

We can also connect better by speaking honestly but without cruelty. For example, we can learn to avoid self-censoring and to have the courage to say what we think and how we feel, rather than keeping quiet or being polite. Indeed, if we aren't straight with each other, we end up with the system that dishonesty deserves.

Also, by encouraging people to speak from the heart, particularly through sharing stories, we discover what matters to people. We bond more strongly and connect with what we hold dear, which is the source of our drive to change. For this reason, it has been said that 'Stories are to transformational change what facts are to Science'.

Open will

In terms of the will, being open means being willing to change.

A significant block to this is the *fear* of change, as witnessed through our safety bias. Getting over fear is a lifelong battle, but we can help the process by fostering our courage, maybe by sticking our necks out in less risky situations and learning how useful this can be and how it makes us more open to change.

Gandhi said 'We must be the change we wish to see in the world'. People who are prepared to change can have a powerful effect in unlocking the courage of others. However, fear makes people demonise those who are trying to change, in an attempt to crush their will. This is done through various forms of abuse ranging from disrespecting them to harassing and bullying them. Many people can withstand a degree of disrespect, but sustained harassment is toxic and can prevent many initiatives that would help us all, from ever seeing the light of day. Again, we could remove these blocks by recognising these tendencies in others as well as in ourselves, and taking a stand against them.

Our collective resolve can be further enhanced if we also encourage our colleagues to speak out against the barriers to progress when they see them, such as unhelpful bias, unfairness or prejudice. Such adverse behaviour isn't just due to people's attitudes, it also flourishes when the situation is against us. For example, if we are under too much pressure or don't give ourselves enough time to consider the options and implications. These can bring out the worst in us. As leaders, we can harness our willingness to change more effectively by reducing the stress where we can, giving people time to discuss and when decisions are proposed, an opportunity to sleep on it.

In summary, if we can reduce the way we block thoughts, people and the attempts at change, we can allow the waters of collaboration to flow more freely and help people to feel more connected to us and to each other.

Being more We than I

> We must choose either to walk in the light of creative altruism or in the darkness of destructive selfishness.
>
> **Martin Luther King Jr**

Not parading our status and sharing our vulnerability says, 'I'm not above you'. Being fair and open-minded says, 'I respect you'. Beyond this, altruism says, 'You, not I, are my main concern'. Mankind may not be capable of complete selflessness but whether or not we believe in altruism, we can still be outward-facing even if we are inward-serving.

Our orientation between I and We is a lifelong issue and it appears that the more our interest becomes outward-facing, the more engaged and connected our colleagues and community become with us. To challenge ourselves, here are a couple of thoughts:

- Isn't ego a force for good? After all, look what can be achieved through competition that rewards individuals.
- Think about a self-oriented leader and an outward-facing one that you've worked with. Which approach got the best from others? Which approach achieved more? What do you make of that?

Self-orientation

Throughout our lives, we are orientated both towards ourselves and towards others. Life experience affects the balance, but people are concerned if our motives as leaders appear to be persistently more to do with self-interest than the interests of others in the team. Why might this be?

This concern makes sense because confidence and connection are needed wherever people are at significant risk. When we are leading some venture, the team may be putting themselves at risk for example from the extra effort involved, the turbulence caused to their lives or the possibility of things going wrong and jobs being affected or lost. These are important matters and people feel much more uneasy and lacking in confidence if they aren't convinced that we are taking notice of their concerns and prioritising their interests.

Over-riding self-interest can also make us selfish, leading to a lack of concern for others, for example in failing to give them adequate time, resources or rewards. Being too self-oriented and 'not having their back' undermines people's trust in us more than most other factors.

Ego

Ego can be an issue, but we shouldn't feel guilty about it because it is natural and it has its uses. For instance, ego can energise us and drive us to achieve. We also need it to help build our self-confidence, self-esteem and personal fortitude. Ego isn't intrinsically bad, but if overplayed it can get in the way of working together with generosity and confidence, as illustrated in the table below. Our ego demands attention but one way of keeping it in check is to 'feed' it in other ways, especially outside work, so that we can collaborate rather more than compete, with our workplace colleagues.

With life experience, the ego can become less needy as the struggle for attention diminishes but this process can't be rushed and for many, our life can't predominantly be about 'We' until it's been sufficiently about 'Me', perhaps to build self-belief. And that's okay.

There comes a point though, as the Martin Luther King Jr quote indicates, where we can choose to be selfish even though there is no longer the need to do so, or move on with our lives by keeping the ego balanced rather than dominant. 'Balance' is an important point because the intention is not to deny the ego. With experience and intent, we can use the power of the ego, for example its drive, whilst not allowing it to inhibit our ability to put the needs of the community first, work well with others, nurture their potential or show our vulnerability.

I	WE
THINKING AS A COMPETITOR	THINKING AS A COLLABORATOR
What is best for me? Will I get the recognition or reward? If other people are better than me, I'll find a way of pretending they are not in order to preserve my self-esteem.	What is best for the community? Where are other people strong and how might we make use of that? How can I give the best of me to our work together? What we achieve together is more important than who gets the credit.

Not everybody instinctively feels a strong sense of connection with the 'We' and we shouldn't feel bad about that even though we may feel pressure to develop that attachment.

Whatever emotional connection we have with the 'We' can be recognised and used. If it isn't strong within us, we can nurture it by keeping an open mind and, as we try to put others first, take notice of how this changes the way people are with us and what can be achieved together. Once we see and feel the benefits, it's possible that the desire for more 'We' and less 'I' will grow and become a powerful and self-perpetuating drive.

Importantly, we mustn't fake what we feel or where we are on our life journey; few things undermine leadership so completely. Because we invest so much in our identity, letting go of our previous selves is painful, even if it is done in anticipation of a better future. However, the kindness of others, encouraged by our honesty, can be a great help.

Our appreciation of others

Leadership, especially at the outset, can make us feel not only valuable but important. We might believe that because we're taking on a burden for the team and putting a lot of effort in, the rewards and status are justified. Or are they?

With leadership, and indeed life experience, we might come to recognise, if we are honest with ourselves, two very significant and related things: first, that we are not as important as we like to believe we are and, second, that others are far more capable than they believe themselves to be. This realisation can challenge our self-perception and our feelings of self-worth.

It is humbling to appreciate that so much of what differentiates people who are given higher or lower status by society is not determined for example by genetics or talent, but by resources, opportunity and support. That isn't to undervalue hard work and ambition, but many people who have been favoured in life have succeeded because of the sacrifice of others who believed in them, such as their parents and teachers. So, how might that insight affect our attitude to others in the team?

Let us consider humility, which is such an important attribute not just of admirable leaders but also of effective ones. The word comes from the Latin humilis meaning 'low' and suggests that such leaders have a low view of their importance. This doesn't mean that they lack confidence or ability, but ties in with the realisation that 'alone I can do so little but together, we can do so much'. In other words, *everyone* is important to the process of change.

Humility, which is not a grudging acknowledgement of the contribution of others, but a more enlightened appreciation of its necessity, helps us see ourselves in a less exalted and more balanced way. It is not easily won as it requires us to step down from our inner pedestal, appreciate rather than just acknowledge the strengths of others, and learn from being vulnerable. This not only teaches humility but also fosters our compassion, as through it we learn what vulnerability might feel like to others in the team, most of whom will not have the shelter of the power and authority that protect our own vulnerability.

Humility teaches us to be human and fallible and not to pretend to be what we are not. Perhaps contrary to our expectations, this is not a diminishing process but an elevating one as through it we learn to respect each other more.

There's a practical edge to appreciating others, too. As leaders, however gifted and committed we are, we can only see the world from one viewpoint and bring but one set of incomplete and often flawed, skills. Our role can never be about personally solving problems, as generally, only a group can do that. The upshot of this is that once we understand that and appreciate the talents of others, we will create opportunities and provide support for them to contribute in a way that self-orientation would *not* drive us to do.

Compassion and caring

The importance of compassion and caring is very clear from the evidence of what makes teams effective. Our team will not connect with us and be motivated to assist, if they feel that we see them as a number rather than as a person.

Effective leaders feel enthused and motivated both of which provide assistance with and protection from, the challenges of change. We therefore need to remind ourselves that for many people, change is felt as pain and effort. Through our compassion, we can acknowledge the difficulties that people have and show that we recognise and care about how they struggle.

Our compassion can also extend beyond individuals and as leaders, we can apply our compassion to the system, constructing the policies and protocols that affect people's lives in ways that are not only fair but humane.

In summary, if we can nurture our sense of 'We' and allow the 'I' to settle and find its place, we can increasingly sense what's good for 'We' and facilitate the changes that bring that about.

Over the stile

Leaders are only leaders if others choose to be influenced by us. Gaining the trust and confidence of others through our integrity and our competence does not come through glittering acts, but through our persistent attempts to deliver whilst living ethically and honestly. This way of living also gives us the securest foundation for our self-belief.

By connecting with people through reducing the status-gap, showing that we need them and making their needs our prime concern, we can create strong relationships that help the community to move forward.

From this foundation, we can cross the stile and safely consider our unique selves, knowing that this is not with the intention of promoting the ego.

In the next chapter we look at what makes each of us different and how using this knowledge makes us more valuable to others, because we are acting in the interests of We, not I.

References

1. Luft, J. & Ingham, H. (1955). The Johari window, a graphic model of interpersonal awareness. *Proceedings of the Western Training Laboratory in Group Development.* Los Angeles: University of California.
2. Greenwald, A., Banaji, M., & Nosek, B. (2011). Project implicit. https://implicit. harvard.edu/implicit/takeatest.html. Accessed 19 November 2019.
3. Scharmer, O. (2016). *Theory U: Leading from the Future as It Emerges* (2nd ed.). Dreamscape Media. ISBN-13: 978-1626567986.

5

Play to your strengths

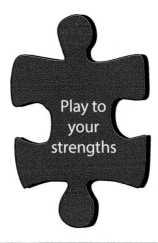

In this chapter, we will explore these questions:

- What are our strengths and why aren't we more aware of them?
- What is it that drives us and how could we connect with it better?
- How can we become stronger by combining what we are naturally talented at?
- How could we use the way we are naturally inclined to think, feel and behave?
- How do others react to our power and how could we use that power more wisely?

All of the jigsaw pieces are important, but this is the longest to discuss. Don't worry, it's not that the topic is difficult, just more extensive, so we will divide this chapter up into four different perspectives on the strongest influences that we have and how we can use them to make us more helpful leaders.

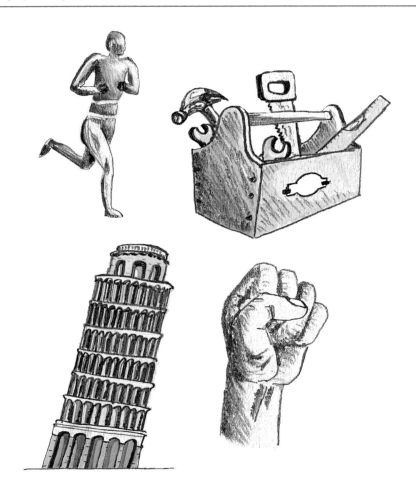

Introduction

Our strengths are those aspects of ourselves that either have or could have significant positive influence on how we work together as a team to improve our situation.

Where are our strengths applied? As leaders, we don't just have a role overseeing the work of the team. We also help it to develop and are usually part of the workforce that carries through its tasks. In addition, there may be other leaders in the organisation under whose guidance we also work, which makes us not only leaders but followers, too. Understanding our strengths helps us to perform better in all these roles.

People often take on a role and later find out where their strengths lie. Instead of this, or in addition to it, we could learn where and how we are most effective (our strengths) and make use of these by tailoring ourselves to the existing situation and by finding new situations that better suit our strengths.

Let's consider an insight about 'strength' which is potentially game-changing for our leadership development. It turns out that our greatest potential for developing our most useful contribution lies not in the areas where we are weak, but in the areas where we are already strong (1).

This seems quite at odds with what we are normally told, for example, in our appraisals, where we are patted on the back for areas of strength and told to 'keep it up' and then advised to turn our efforts to working harder on our deficiencies.

There's a caveat here, which is that we can't ignore incompetence; playing to our strengths is not an excuse for ignoring our potentially dangerous weaknesses. We need to be 'good enough' all-rounders in the areas that matter, especially amongst our skills. Significantly poor performance, for example in our communication or technical skills, can't be left unaddressed.

However, beyond taking action so that we maintain our overall competence, the evidence suggests that we should direct our time and effort to areas where we are already talented and seek to make these outstanding, not just for ourselves but because this is how we can maximise our benefit to the team. This principle doesn't just apply to leaders of course, it applies to everyone.

Case example

Chen is a young manager who is naturally good at listening, calming people down and helping them to find a way forward. He builds on this by going on a conflict resolution course and is now able to apply this skill in the practice, where he spots disputes early and helps people work though disagreements. The time, emotional distress and cost he saves the team through being proactive and skilled, is invaluable to them.

What are the sources of our strengths?

In this chapter, we don't pretend to be all-inclusive and for simplicity we will illustrate our strengths in four domains. These are what we are most *driven* by, our strongest *skills*, our most useful biases and *inclinations* and where we have *power* to influence positively.

The strengths that arise from each of these domains can make our influence more beneficial to the team. For example:

- A strong *drive* for fairness can help a team improve morale and productivity.
- Strong *skills* can help teams to think better, relate better and complete tasks more effectively.

- A strong personality *inclination*, for example towards being extroverted may keep the team energised, or toward introversion could encourage the group to consider issues more deeply.

- A strong *power* that others feel from us and which has an influence on the way they think, feel and behave. For example, the power that arises from being respected for our values, which might help a team to take the moral dimension of problems more seriously. This, by the way, is a great example of what we mean by having power *through* people, rather than *over* them.

Our strengths reflect something about our deeper dispositions. Rather than just being areas in which we can train ourselves to be better, they reflect ways in which we naturally 'are'. For example, areas in which we are talented, gifted or where our skills come naturally and easily. Because they are deep-seated and may seem innate, we are usually only subconsciously aware of them as strengths, which is why they are often underused or at times, badly used. Such strengths may, however, be more obvious to others.

Being naturally strong in an area means that our *influence* there is also potentially strong. However, that does not mean that our influence is necessarily effective or useful to the team. In fact, strengths can be toxic if overdone so we have to learn to tailor ourselves and apply our strengths at the appropriate time and place and to the appropriate degree. This becomes possible as we learn to recognise our strengths, to knowingly use them and to bring them together so that they complement each other.

Don't feel limited by the way we have split up different sources of strength. Overall, do you have a sense of where your natural talent lies, what others say you are really good at or where they say they particularly value what you bring? This is what you should make more use of.

Using our strengths also *feels* good because it resonates and makes us feel we are in our 'flow'. This is a really important feeling to recognise, because it signals where we are strong, where our potentially greatest contribution lies and where we could, or even should, be investing more of our lives. Beyond our own strengths, as leaders we have an invaluable opportunity to help others to discover *their* strengths and to provide opportunities for these to be amplified and applied.

The process of developing strengths is potentially disruptive, although in a good way. It needs to be managed because, for example, as people develop, they may move on to different roles or occasionally, move out to other organisations if they outgrow ours. As leaders, we would not view these outcomes negatively but see them as being signs of growth and therefore of success.

Let's now consider each of these dimensions of our strengths.

Harness your drives

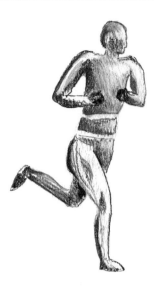

What are they?

Drives are our fuel. They are a major source of our energy, the force that powers us, and nothing can be changed or achieved without them, both in leadership and in life more generally.

We recognise them through how they energise us, although we may not always know where they come from. Feeling the drive, the energy from within, can sometimes be the first clue that something that matters to us, needs our attention. Our drives take us on a journey by both initiating and supporting it through the long and often tedious process of change so that we don't give up or give in. The following is an example of this.

Case example

Christine was a new partner in a partnership of six that hadn't changed for over ten years. Because the partners worked at two sites, they didn't get together each day and Christine felt isolated as a result.

She had a strong desire to develop relationships and feel that she 'belonged' and because this wasn't being met, she was unhappy. She also believed that others in the team were suffering for the same reason and this created a strong drive to do something about it.

(Continued)

The manager and some partners were very resistant to her idea that they should get together for a coffee break after surgery and many practical problems were thrown in her way. It took three years, but now the break is seen as invaluable and has improved communication, support and morale not just for Christine but for the whole team.

How do we become aware of our drives?

Here are three techniques that help us to become aware of our drives:

1   Self-awareness helps us to notice the feeling of energy and propulsion that our drives create in us and which make us want to *do* something. They make us want to move from here, where we feel uncomfortable, unhappy or dissatisfied to there, which we believe to be a better place.

   At a deeper level, our drives reflect our dispositions to, for example, be kind, fight injustice, learn, enthuse, enable, see the problems and so on. Because they are deep-level, many of these also reflect what we are inspired by, especially when we see them in others. As we noted in Chapter 3, our inspiration is particularly noteworthy because it is a potent source of our energy.

2   Another way is to reflect on ourselves, perhaps guided by a model. This may sound a bit theoretical but it needn't be abstract as it can uncover thoughts and feelings that already lie within. To give you an idea, here's an example of a model from Kahler (2) in which five drivers are described, that many find easy to relate to. Excerpts from this model are shown below; these help us to recognise our dominant drive and see how the positives that it identifies can be used to benefit our teamwork.

   Strong drives can be overplayed and we can see through the 'drawbacks' column how, if this happened, it could cause stress and unhappiness in ourselves and in other people. However, help is at hand and some ways of keeping our strengths in balance are shown in the last column.

DRIVER	POSITIVES	DRAWBACKS	HOW TO AVOID THE DRAWBACKS
Be Perfect	I produce accurate, reliable work	I have a fear of failure I tend to criticise those who are less than perfect	Learn to laugh at my mistakes Learn to be happy with producing work that isn't perfect but is 'good enough'
Be Strong	I tend to stay calm I like to take control	I don't like to ask for help I can be seen as aggressive or unfeeling	Learn where my strength can feel threatening to others and then try to connect with people better Learn that it's okay to have feelings
Hurry Up	I like to do everything quickly I thrive on getting lots done	I make mistakes because I'm rushing I get agitated with those who are slower than me (most people)	Learn to pause and think before acting Recognise my irritation but remind myself that I'm the odd one out, not them
Please Others	I'm always checking that people are happy with me and my work	I avoid conflict and am reluctant to challenge other people when I need to I tend to take criticism personally; to me, criticism always hurts	Learn to be more self-confident and self-sufficient Learn to accept criticism without feeling a failure
Try Hard	I'm enthusiastic and help get things started	I'm never satisfied I get tense and anxious	Don't move to another task until the first is completed

Which of these drives do you feel strongly within yourself? Has this drive caused you problems? If so, could you make use of any of the suggestions in the table?

Let's pause for a moment and consider the drive called 'Be strong', itself a feeling or drive that many leaders have. This incorporates the desire for power, which we will discuss later. This desire is like a drug, so if it's part of our makeup we should bear in mind that it's healthy in small doses where it can make us bolder, but toxic if there's too much, when it could lead to bullying others or to the desire to win even at their expense.

3   We all learn in different ways and, for some, tools such as online questionnaires can help us to clarify where we are strong and can offer advice on how to make the most of this in our leadership. The 'Insight into Action' questionnaire, which helps clarify our strongest drives and skills is an example (3).

Where do our drives come from?

Let's consider three aspects of this and how we can apply what we learn to ourselves and our teams.

*   *Intrinsic and extrinsic motives*

    Actions often have reasons for them, which if we are aware of, we call motives. It is helpful to consider them as follows:

    Extrinsic is the motivation to perform an activity to earn a reward or to avoid a punishment, both of these being 'external' to ourselves. Common external motivators include wealth, reputation, status and regulation.

    Intrinsic arises from within us and is something we don't do for external reasons but because we find it pleasurable or fulfilling (like writing a book?).

    Both extrinsic and intrinsic motivation are powerful, one is not 'better' and they can coexist with each having its time and place. Extrinsic motivation can help us get started, give us a reason to take on something we may not otherwise be driven to do and can also help us develop new perspectives and skills that we may not have otherwise gained.

However, intrinsic motivation may ultimately feel more meaningful, particularly in the health service where many people have a strong sense of values, belief and vocation. Intrinsic motivation resonates with what matters to us personally, and because of this it has the power to keep us going, especially when things get difficult.

- *Desire for autonomy mastery and purpose*

  These are big ideas, but let's use a very simple example. If you've ever learned to drive a car, you'll remember how it felt to be given the keys and be allowed to sit in the driving seat and take charge. This is *autonomy*. At another level, there might have been more satisfaction from, at the umpteenth attempt, *mastering* the art of parallel parking. Lastly, there might have been the greatest satisfaction of all from putting the driving skills to good *purpose*, for instance to gain personal freedom in a remote area or even to drive an ambulance and use that skill to do something meaningful for the community.

  Can you imagine how we could use this progression to create opportunities that engage and motivate our team? We've given only a short paragraph to this, but motivation is a really important topic that we will revisit in Chapter 14.

- *Our deeper needs*

  Our human needs lie deep and because we feel them rather more than understand them, we will explore that understanding here. As an example of human needs, we have the desire to be accepted and not to disappoint others and this drives many of us to work hard so as to avoid guilt. Sound familiar?

  People sometimes feel that they shouldn't have drives like guilt or ambition, but there is nothing intrinsically good or bad about these. The fuel is less important than where we are going with it and perhaps more significant is that if we can accept the way we are and use our drives well, they can energise and motivate us.

Our drives lead to action and to visualise the connection, take a look at the diagram below. On the left is Maslow's model (4) of a proposed hierarchy of human needs which we've shown because it is intuitive to many and is widely used. The dotted line in the diagram represents the threshold of consciousness and we can see how subconscious needs can initially be perceived as feelings and can then surface as conscious motives. The motives that we feel can then address the subconscious needs by converting them to actions.

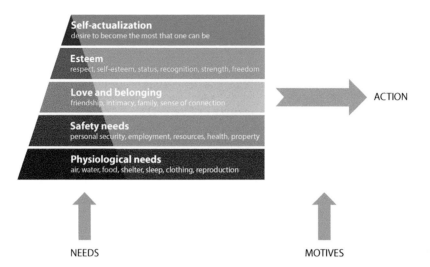

We should point out that Maslow's suggestion of a hierarchy and a natural progression through them is contested as it has a number of difficulties. For instance, it isn't proven that the natural flow through life is from bottom to top as represented by Maslow. Also, it isn't the case that some needs are more important than others, that everyone has the same hierarchy or that different cultures agree on which needs are more valued than others. As an example, for some people and cultures, the social needs and responsibilities of 'love and belonging' are the pinnacle, rather than achieving personal fulfilment through 'self-actualisation' as advocated in those societies that champion the autonomy of the individual.

Nevertheless, it's a memorable way of picturing an important but hidden part of ourselves in a way that stimulates our thinking and helps us make sense of ourselves. For instance, it might suggest the notion that all needs are potentially important to individuals and to healthy societies and that a balance between them may be desirable.

Also, it might suggest that the degree of personal need in each of these areas differs between us, and that this might affect our behaviour and aptitude. For instance, some suggest that managers or assessors who are required at times to be ruthless may be more successful if they have a low absolute need for 'love and belonging' from the team.

The relative demand between our needs also varies over time as might the possibility of meeting them. For example, for those who achieve some self-actualisation, this usually comes through many years of life experience and learning. Likewise, it takes a good deal of investing in relationships in a community, thereby meeting our 'belonging' need, before we can earn the recognition and respect from them that helps us meet our 'esteem' need.

So, how could we visualise these needs and their associated motives, leading to action in the real world? Here's an example from practice life.

Case example

Nicola is a newly qualified nurse who has recently been promoted and is joining the practice nursing team. Although she is well qualified, she is inexperienced compared to the other nurses who are significantly older. She feels unsettled because she is anxious to be seen to be 'up to the mark' by her peers and she wants to feel accepted by the nursing team.

We can see that Nicola has a couple of basic human needs. The first is a 'safety need'. She is anxious about making a mistake and she addresses this by asking for all her consultations to be checked and debriefed in her first week. She knows this isn't sustainable long-term but it allows her to develop her confidence and to be seen to be willing to learn.

She addresses her second need, which is to 'belong' or feel part of the team, by trying to get to know more about her colleagues' home lives, and by sharing stories and pictures from her own.

In summary, the important thing is that by recognising the drives that come from our human needs, we can harness their energy and attend to our needs more knowingly. In so doing, we can not only feel better in ourselves and do better for others, but we can help ourselves to grow and mature.

In this section, these insights on our drives help us to connect with our subconscious selves. We may want to reflect on the drive that makes us take on leadership in the first place. The models that we have used are not exhaustive, but they give us a way of harnessing our drives better and helping our colleagues when they appear unhappy and disconnected from what drives *them*.

Getting our needs met here and elsewhere

Because our needs are powerful and persistent drivers, they'll insist on being addressed to some degree, but it matters where we do that. Why might that be?

Using the divide between work and home as an example, if we don't get a need sufficiently satisfied in one context, the burden may end up being met in the other.

To get an appreciation of this, think of your desires for power and control, affirmation and importance, intimacy and delight. These are important and almost universal desires, so are they sufficiently satisfied? Is the balance between the places in which they are met, appropriate?

For instance, if we have fallen out with our partner at home and feel unloved, we might seek to rectify that at work. Alternatively, if we lack sufficient control at work, we may overdominate at home and so on. In their own ways, both over-reactions could be inappropriate and dangerous and because they are subconsciously driven, we may not recognise what we are doing, and why, at an early enough stage.

One way of avoiding this is to use our insight and our ability to plan, to address our basic needs before they become a problem. Such needs include feeling some sense of control, feeling valued and feeling affection. These need to be satisfied frequently, possibly daily, and therefore nearby. They are best not 'stored up' to deal with when we have the time. For these reasons, it is worth reflecting on these needs, where and when they are met and whether the balance is healthy.

Nurture your strongest skills

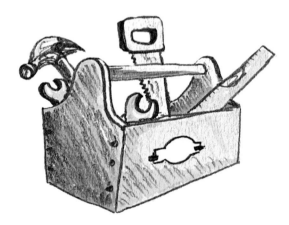

How do our skills connect with our drives?

We've discussed how our drives are the fuel that energises us to move forward, but this energy will do no good if it isn't *applied* effectively. This is where our skills come in, which we can think of as attributes that are not necessarily innate but can be developed through training. This is liberating because it opens up the possibility of competent leadership to all those who have the opportunity and the will to learn. Perhaps this is why we could suggest that good leaders are more made than born.

Drive and skill need each other, but why is this? As leaders, if we had high drive but low skills, our team may buy into the issue and be willing to support change, spurred on by the energy of our drive. However, our lack of leadership skills and therefore lack of competence could doom the project to failure.

On the other hand, suppose we had high skills but poor drive? In that instance, people may not come on board in the first place because our lack of drive and passion had failed to generate sufficient concern, interest and momentum. It's like boarding a train that has no engine. You wouldn't do it and expect to go anywhere.

Skills and the 'primary colours of leadership'

'Primary colours' is a wonderfully simple and intuitive model of leadership (5) shown in the diagram below that neatly illustrates the range of skills and how they overlap. Its simplicity means that we can draw ideas from it at a number of levels in ways that deepen our understanding. For instance, because this chapter is about our personal aptitudes, we apply the model here to ourselves as individuals. However, the model could also be applied at the level of a team or even a larger community, showing how the range of skills discussed below are also applicable to groups of people engaged in common endeavours.

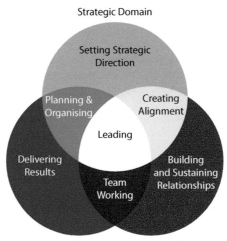

The primary colours of leadership are green, red and blue, and we could think of these as 'Thinking' skills, 'Relating to people' skills and 'Management' skills, respectively. Put even more simply, we can think of head, heart and hands.

Leadership is about change and if change is to happen effectively, efficiently and with the least unnecessary suffering for the people in our organisation, all three colours need to be well-represented. The most effective leaders use the skills in which they are particularly strong, but they do not pretend to be gifted in all areas and therefore do not attempt to be self-sufficient.

Instead, they identify where the skills lie across the team, orchestrate them by bringing them in at the right time and place and through this process, lead the team to success. However, they can't do that if people's skills are not known, available or developed to a high enough standard in the first place. Taking this global view and finding out what people are strong at, developing strengths in *all* the colours across the team rather than in each individual, and then making use of them by design rather than by chance, is a holy grail in leadership.

As individuals, we are each gifted in different ways and the evidence shows that no effective leader is a strong performer in all three colours. Generally, we have a natural strength in one, we are pretty good in another and the third we may have to work around. We 'work around' partly by using our other skills to compensate but more especially by bringing in other people to complement our strengths by applying their strengths to areas in which we are weak.

Working around is reassuring as it gives us permission to be human and not feel bad about our weaknesses. By recognising that we cannot go it alone, it also helps us to respect the strength in others and to value diversity. The flip side of this insight is the realisation that the team needs us to make more use of *our* natural skill strength, which we call our 'primary colour'.

Which is your primary colour: head, heart or hands?

- Reflecting on what you know about yourself rather than on what other people or your role expect you to be, have a think about these colours. You will have them all, of course, but which is the one that feels the strongest and comes the most easily?
- Which is your least natural, and if you compensate for that, how do you do it? If you don't, what does that say? There's more on this in Chapter 7.
- If you think you are equally strong in all colours, you may be fooling yourself and diverting energy away from where your strongest contribution lies.

Head

Are you someone who principally loves to think about problems and issues, perhaps interpreting the data, reading articles or networking with people to find out what happens elsewhere? Are you driven to understand and learn? Do you like the world of ideas, or perhaps enjoy dreaming, using your imagination and conceptualising a better future? If so, your primary colour is Green. You are a 'head' person. That doesn't mean you are necessarily exceptionally bright or intellectual, just that you are instinctively drawn to the head stuff of knowledge, understanding and imagination.

Heart

Perhaps it's the people who interest you most, how they are feeling and what their thoughts and concerns might be? You might be principally interested in relationships, how to understand and connect with people and how to be together more happily and perhaps more productively. When something is proposed, your first thought might be about how it would affect the lives of the team or of particular individuals. You might be keen to see people develop and to get the best out of them. If so, your primary colour is Red. You are a relationship or 'heart' person.

Hands

Maybe your interest is more about the process. That doesn't mean that you don't have ideas or dreams or that you don't care about the people; far from it, but it may be that you get most engaged when you are thinking about how to convert a plan into action; actually *do* something. When an idea is discussed you can immediately see what needs to happen to make practical use of it, who needs to be involved, when and how. Although vision is important and you don't disrespect that, you really want to get things done, so people are not wasting their time. Does this sound like you? If so, then your primary colour is Blue. You are a practical or 'hands-on' person.

Can you think of people known to you who exemplify each of these colours?

Now that you know your primary colour, you can stop wasting your life on 'correcting' your weaknesses but instead work around them. They are weaknesses because you are just not naturally good at them, unlike your primary colour, which is where you are naturally gifted.

Different 'tribes' such as groups of colleagues, teams and organisations value some colours over others and, as leaders, we need to appreciate where this happens and compensate for it.

For example, a technical team may value the head but may not think that the relationships are important. This could significantly damage the team's effectiveness and as leaders we could anticipate this and take corrective action.

Importantly, we need to create a team culture in which all colours are seen as essential and no one feels that their area of strength is a poor relation in the mix.

Developing our range of skills through mixing the colours

Now that we've identified our natural skill strength, we can look to see how to make it even more effective. One powerful way is making dominant use of it but using it in combination with its neighbouring colour. These overlaps are shown in the diagram, and the skills that arise and which are important to leadership are described in the table shown below. Because we are building our overlap from the foundation of our natural area of strength, the new skills described could be developed to a high standard.

OVERLAP AND SKILL	COMMENT (SKILLS ARE IN ITALICS)
Green and Red, *Creating alignment*	The green 'head' skills of problem-solving and coming up with ideas combines with the red world of relating to people. Creating alignment equips us as leaders to *explain, discuss, get people on board, elicit their ideas* and help everyone shift position so that they, and we, see more eye to eye.
Red and Blue *Team working*	The red skills of connecting with people, identifying what they are good at and creating opportunities for them to contribute, joins the blue world of 'getting stuff done'. As a result, we can 'team-work', which in this model is not the cosy exercise of being nice to people and making them cups of tea, but the challenging work of *keeping people to task, getting them to deliver what they said they would, supporting them if in need of help and stretching them* if they are coasting, so that they can develop and become even more capable.
Green and Blue, *Planning and organising*	The blue hands-on world of managing, combines with the green world of thinking ahead. In so doing, we can *anticipate what the future might hold and make plans that clarify the way ahead and avoid the pitfalls* that we are aware of. Planning also helps us to *develop timelines and identify milestones* which between them mark the way, maintain motivation or give an early sign that we are off-pace or even off-track. '*Organising*' skills do what they say on the tin, and help us be more efficient, effective and thereby give the team a feeling of confidence and purpose.

Let's take a practical example. Suppose that our dominant colour is green, meaning that we are a 'head' person, driven principally to think. To use this strength to its greatest effect, we need to combine it with the red (relationship) domain on one side and the blue domain (hands-on planning and organising) on the other:

Case example

- Ed is a green person who loves the ideas but lives in his own head. He prefers the written word but recognises that he could be a lot more effective if he came out from behind his desk and communicated more. Ed does this and in so doing, finds that dialogue helps him to get people on board, challenge his mindset and as a result, come up with better ideas.
- Ed also teams up with Karen, who is a natural communicator. She is good with people, amusing and is able to take Ed's work and present it well. They try working as a double-act in a meeting and it goes down well, with Ed getting extra credit from the team for coming out of his comfort zone and engaging with people directly.
- In these two ways, Ed takes his natural strength in green and makes it even more effective by combining with the red domain.
- He also tries combining with the blue domain and does this by planning and organising a workshop that takes ideas, for example on how to use health apps as part of chronic disease management, and applies them to practical situations.
- Hence, by combining with red, Ed finds that his ideas are discussed and improved. By combining with blue, Ed finds that the ideas can be implemented successfully and used to make a practical difference to patient care.

This example shows that our natural skill strength, as seen through our dominant colour, is not maximised by using it in isolation but by combining it with its adjoining colours. This insight helps individuals but, even more significantly, helps teams to be more effective.

Using the strength of our consulting skills

Consulting skills are not part of the professional experience of every leader, but for those that have them, they offer a range of tools that could enhance our leadership.

For clinicians, in the consultation, we use the care we feel for people to help us approach a problem, negotiate a plan and help the patient find a way forward despite anxiety, uncertainty and risk. Leadership in some ways is like consulting but at a bigger scale, and consulting skills are transferable to the world beyond the consulting room door – and vice versa.

To illustrate this simply, let's artificially split some skills into those relating to 'people' and others to 'task'. In the figures below, we list skills that we primarily use in the consulting room and, separately, beyond the consulting room door, we list skills that are related but are used in the wider community.

Taking people skills first:

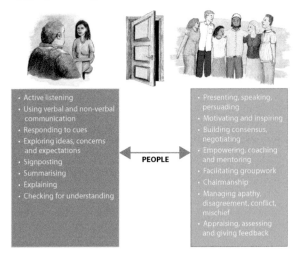

- Active listening
- Using verbal and non-verbal communication
- Responding to cues
- Exploring ideas, concerns and expectations
- Signposting
- Summarising
- Explaining
- Checking for understanding

PEOPLE

- Presenting, speaking, persuading
- Motivating and inspiring
- Building consensus, negotiating
- Empowering, coaching and mentoring
- Facilitating groupwork
- Chairmanship
- Managing apathy, disagreement, conflict, mischief
- Appraising, assessing and giving feedback

As we will see in Chapter 20, many 'people' skills from the consultation can help us to chair more effectively. Likewise, the coaching skills that we develop with colleagues outside the consulting room could be applied to help patients alter their lifestyle.

Looking at the 'Task' skills:

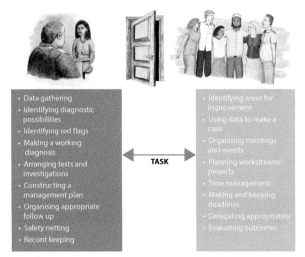

- Data gathering
- Identifying diagnostic possibilities
- Identifying red flags
- Making a working diagnosis
- Arranging tests and investigations
- Constructing a management plan
- Organising appropriate follow up
- Safety netting
- Record keeping

TASK

- Identifying areas for improvement
- Using data to make a case
- Organising meetings and events
- Planning workstreams/ projects
- Time management
- Making and keeping deadlines
- Delegating appropriately
- Evaluating outcomes

Let's take the consultation skill of explaining the risks and benefit of treatment to patients. Applying this to the wider world, when we try to persuade people to change, we can employ facts, diagrams and well-presented information to 'use data to make a case'.

In the other direction, 'time management' and 'keeping deadlines' through prioritising, setting manageable goals, managing expectations and so on can give us better control back in the consulting room, even if it cannot guarantee that we run to time.

This brief illustration shows us the potential of using consulting skills, with which we may be very familiar, to help ourselves and others to become more effective leaders.

Undiscovered strengths

How do we become aware of our undiscovered strengths, areas in which we may be talented without realising? It's worth experimenting and trying out different activities that aren't usual for us. We may find from what people say about us or from how we find ourselves mastering something quickly, that we have a talent that we hadn't suspected, for example, for such things as humour, public speaking, writing, enthusing or teaching people. Another method is to try asking colleagues, 'What am I the "go to" person for?' The great thing is that whatever our talent, there will be a way of bringing it in to our work and using it to make our leadership and teamworking more effective.

Case example

Craig is a GP partner and is the lead on financial matters and issues to do with the premises. This is dry stuff, but Craig can sing well and does so at practice functions including the Christmas party. Rather than having a reputation for being boring because of his lead roles, it's amazing how much people warm to him because of how he entertains them socially. The team is a better place because of it.

Adapt to your inclinations

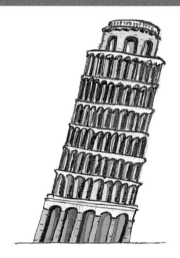

In addition to the prejudices and negative biases that we discussed in Chapter 4 and which threaten the trust and confidence that others have in us, we have more benign inclinations that reflect our preferences and the ways we like to behave. We can get a sense of these through reflection and feedback and both these techniques remain the cornerstone of self-awareness.

However, it can also be helpful to use the psychometric tools which have been developed for the purpose. These tools probe sensitive areas like our aptitudes, identity and beliefs and shed light on the 'unknown unknowns', which are those aspects of ourselves that we are not aware of and others are also not aware of and can't therefore give feedback about. The real value of these tools comes from discussing the results with colleagues who can give us a sense of balance and perspective.

Let's consider two examples of such tools and how they might be used to identify our preferences. These preferences, once known and employed, are another manifestation of where we are strong.

Belbin Role inventory

The first is the Belbin Role inventory (6) which is a powerful tool for identifying personal role preferences and the mix across the team, based on a questionnaire. Some teams use it to identify role gaps so that these can inform recruitment decisions. Others use it to see whether people are in the jobs that best suit their role-preferences. Applied to ourselves, if the results suggest that we are in an appropriate role, then we can be reassured that our area of strength is being well-employed. If not, we may need to consider whether, for the sake of the team as well as ourselves, we need to modify our role.

Just as we did earlier when we looked at our overlapping skill colours, we can improve our 'role-strength' by working on it, as well as with it. How could we do this? Take a look at the final column in the table that follows. If weaknesses are 'allowable', that does not mean that they are unchangeable, so try and imagine how they could be modified. Here's an example:

Case example

Penny, a junior GP partner, finds from the Belbin inventory that she is a 'shaper'. Her qualities are vital to the team as she is not reticent about holding employees to account and pushing them to keep their commitments. She is fairly thick-skinned and admits that one of the allowable weaknesses, 'offending people's feelings', applies to her.

To become more effective in her area of strength, she undertakes communication skills training so that she can pick up on body language more proficiently and learn to listen and empathise better. She gets good feedback from her colleagues, who support her as they appreciate that this is hard for her. She feels more included in the team and even looks forward to socialising with them, which she has avoided doing in the past.

Because she becomes better at using an area of natural strength, she becomes a better helper and therefore, a better leader in her team.

(*Continued*)

Case example (*Continued*)

Team Role		Contribution	Allowable Weaknesses
Plant		Creative, imaginative, free-thinking. Generates ideas and solves difficult problems.	Ignores incidentals. Too preoccupied to communicate effectively.
Resource Investigator		Outgoing, enthusiastic, communicative. Explores opportunities and develops contacts.	Over-optimistic. Loses interest once initial enthusiasm has passed.
Co-ordinator		Mature, confident, identifies talent. Clarifies goals. Delegates effectively.	Can be seen as manipulative. Offloads own share of the work.
Shaper		Challenging, dynamic, thrives on pressure. Has the drive and courage to overcome obstacles.	Prone to provocation. Offends peoples feelings.
Monitor Evaluator		Sober, strategic and discerning. Sees all options and judges accurately.	Lacks drive and ability to inspire others. Can be overly critical.
Teamworker		Co-operative, perceptive and diplomatic. Listens and averts friction.	Indecisive in crunch situations. Avoids confrontation.
Implementer		Practical, reliable, efficient. Turns ideas into actions and organises work that needs to be done.	Somewhat inflexible. Slow to respond to new possibilities.
Completer Finisher		Painstaking, conscientious, anxious. Searches out errors. Polishes and perfects.	Inclined to worry unduly. Reluctant to delegate.
Specialist		Single-minded, self-starting, dedicated. Provides knowledge and skills in rare supply.	Contributes only on a narrow front. Dwells on technicalities.

Personality analysis

The second example of a tool is of the five personality traits, sometimes known as the 'big five' (7). These are malleable with age and there are questionnaires that can help us understand and interpret our natural dispositions. Their importance relates to a number of factors:

- How these dispositions make us think and behave with other people
- How we can apply the strengths that they signify
- How we can also reduce the shadow these dispositions sometimes cast on those we interact with

Despite our assumptions, there are no good or bad traits and each of them can be a strength. Unfortunately, the names given to the traits are very loaded so don't be put off by them. For instance, as the diagram shows, if we score highly for 'neuroticism', we may initially feel appalled and find it difficult to see how this could be interpreted as a strength and as something useful to society. Yet, as shown, neuroticism gives us an ability to focus, especially on the important minutiae that others get impatient with and overlook. For example, we might pick up on things in the small print that have serious financial implications for the practice, or notice details in the workplace that affect patient safety.

Another common negative reaction is to the realisation that we are introverted rather than extroverted. Introverts get a bad press. However, introverted people are often more reflective and thoughtful, both of which lead to deeper insight and the ability to support people, which are greatly valued by other team members.

So, thank goodness for the neurotics and the introverts. We would be so much poorer without them.

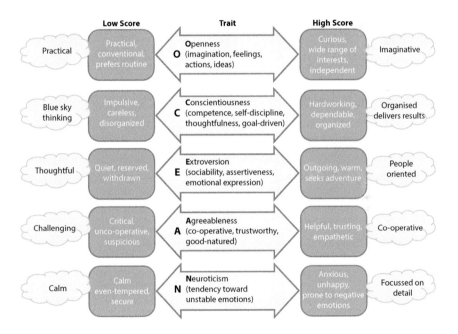

As we discussed in Chapter 4, it is important to be authentic and trust-worthy and not to try to mimic any trait that isn't a natural part of our makeup. That doesn't mean that we shouldn't make full use of the traits that we have even if they are not strong. For example, all leaders need to energise people and if our inclination to 'extroversion' is low, we may need to make the greatest use of what we have to help us energise others.

In addition, those inclinations that are *marked* are potentially part of our strengths if we learn to knowingly put them to constructive use.

Be wise with your power

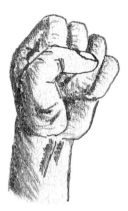

Generally, we should seek to have power through others, not power over others.

The ethics of influence

Influencing people is natural and normal. If we think about it, we can't *not* influence those around us and that fact applies to everyone in the team, leaders and followers alike because we all influence each other all the time. Influence and power are issues for everyone, particularly those who feel they don't have enough of them.

In terms of using it, this is more of an issue for leaders because our personal influence is greater, although it is also the case that people without obvious power and authority have much more influence than they would believe. So, the question is not whether we should or should not use influence, but how we do it in ways that are both effective and socially acceptable.

How do you personally feel about using your influence: perhaps you are uncomfortable with the notion? Well that's good, because leadership, which incorporates the expert use of our positive influence, is a constant challenge to our ethical behaviour and a challenge at both extremes of our influence. Let's consider this in more detail.

The dangers of *overusing* our influence are clear as people may feel coerced into doing something against their will, or feel that they are not valued because their perspective is not being sought or respected. Overusing our influence can also mean that other people's talents are being underused. This can be detrimental as it may stop the team from developing and becoming more capable, hence the saying that 'a leader with an unimpressive team will accomplish unimpressive things'.

However, *underusing* our influence can also be problematic as we may fail to intervene in ways that could facilitate improvement, give confidence to people and prevent unnecessary anxiety and suffering. So, does underusing our influence feel like an ethical problem too? Would it be too much to suggest that at its extreme we might think of 'underuse' as a form of neglect?

We can help ourselves to get the balance right. For example, we can be vigilant and periodically check that others don't find us too forceful or manipulative or at the other extreme, that they don't think of us as being 'absent' when we are needed. At a deeper level, we can use our courage and openness to maintain trust by owning up when we are getting it wrong with our influence and then take steps to get a better balance.

Being aware of our power and using it well

Power is the capacity to influence the attitudes and behaviour of people in a particular direction and it comes from a number of sources, which French and Raven (8) have usefully classified. Because we all have influence, we all have power.

Good leaders know about power and their greatest legacy does not come from the power of control but from how they use their influence to improve the people, including helping them to lead in their own right. Good leaders beget good leaders. The opposite may also be true.

If part of our personal strength is the power that we have, then recognising where this comes from can help us to use it better. To do this, we can try to really notice how people react to us, because through their emotions and behaviour, they are signalling how our power and influence affect them.

Now look at the table, which is based on the theory of the sources of power, bearing in mind that for each of us there will be several ways in which people react to us depending on which sources our power is derived from, who we are working with and what the context is. This table is not all-inclusive.

I NOTICE THAT PEOPLE	WHY MIGHT THIS BE?	HOW COULD I USE THIS INFLUENCE BETTER?
Look up to me	I may have expertise that they don't, possibly clinical, technical or practical.	If overdone, people could feel inadequate, so I could share knowledge, openly recognise the expertise of others and make myself more approachable so that they don't put me on a pedestal, but feel connected to me.
Admire me	People may want to be like me, perhaps because I embody certain values or attitudes that are important to us all.	People clearly identify with me and feel I represent something important about them. I could clarify what this is and speak up for it on behalf of the team.
Fear me	Rather than fearing me personally, they may fear the influential position I hold, which could be as manager, senior partner or someone seen as a 'boss'. It is still possible that there are also aspects of my behaviour that people fear, which are to do with me personally and not my position.	Fear is not helpful, so there are a number of things I can do to help people convert their fear of *me* to respect for the *position*. For instance: <ul><li>I could remember their fear, even anticipate it, and seek to put people at ease where needed.</li><li>I should make sure my requests are appropriate and that I'm not using my power as a lazy way of getting people to do what I want.</li><li>I should make it clear that when I insist on proper procedures, it's not to get back at anyone but to show openness and fairness to all.</li><li>I shouldn't hold back from doing the unpleasant things like getting people to pull their weight, reprimanding them or even punishing them when needed. The wider team lose confidence if these things aren't done.</li></ul>

(Continued)

84

I NOTICE THAT PEOPLE	WHY MIGHT THIS BE?	HOW COULD I USE THIS INFLUENCE BETTER?
		• People fear being punished so I should make sure that rules and penalties are well-known and clear. I should ensure that any punishment is fair, consistent and given in private. • I mustn't forget that because everyone including myself can get it wrong, being forgiving and helping colleagues to rehabilitate is really important. • Although I may not want to believe this possible, I could seek feedback to clarify if there are aspects of me (rather than my role) that make people fearful, and address these.
Wish to please me	I may be in a position to reward them, for example with bonuses, opportunities or resources.	I could make use of the power of giving rewards in order to encourage desired behaviour and action. To maintain this influence and stop it becoming discredited, I should make sure I have a fair and open system, check that people have earned rewards appropriately and that the rewards are what people actually want, not just what I'm prepared to give. Some of the most meaningful rewards of all are recognition, praise and thanks. The best thing about these is that they can be given frequently and for free. Am I doing that enough?
Are in conflict with me	They might find me threatening.	Although there are many causes of conflict, could this be triggered by my (ab)use of power? I may not have remembered or noticed which forms of power I'm using and I could check on this and make any changes that would help me to use my influence better.

If a significant part of our power comes from a role, there are aspects of such positions that may be toxic. Too much 'role power' can distance us from people and stop us caring about them. It can also disconnect us so that we run the risk of becoming disinhibited and rash. Because role power has a historic tradition, not only may we use it but also our colleagues may expect us to do so.

To guard against overuse, we need to stay connected with people, interacting with them frequently enough to pick up on the cues that show us how we are coming across, whether we are using our influence well and whether we are keeping on track.

To stay balanced in our feelings about ourselves and therefore in our dealings with other people, it's important to remind ourselves that we are not (just) our role. We do not have to be defined either by ourselves or by others as the job that we do; as people we are much broader than that. We can also learn not to take things too personally by remembering that we should not mistake criticism of the role, which is inevitable, as being criticism of ourselves as people: easy to say, very hard not to feel, however.

Let's go back to the *underuse* of influence. In the flattened hierarchies we have in primary care, we can see what happens when power is underused. For example, this can lead to people putting up with unnecessarily prolonged and draining debates. Not stepping in when needed can also lead to damaging manoeuvring and to mischievous behaviour. So, here is an important point; using power well does not mean *not* using it.

The table is liberating because we can see how we might make use of these different manifestations of power without relying on any one of them exclusively. Important as they may be, we can also see why we don't need to have a title, status or particular expertise to have the power to influence. As a result, anyone and everyone in the team has a legitimate, and we could argue necessary, influence. In the team, each of us can learn to recognise our influence and use it well and as leaders, we have an important role in helping to make that happen.

We explore 'power' further in Chapter 10.

Putting our strengths together

We are now at the end of the chapter and, to reiterate, we are at our most useful and effective when we make the most of what is best about us and use this in our roles as leaders and as followers.

In the example given here, we consider four strengths that Asha, a reception manager, has become aware of over a long period of working in the team. For the sake of clarity, we have only shown one of the strengths she has in each of the domains and then suggested how she could harness these.

DOMAIN	ASHA'S STRENGTH	HOW COULD ASHA USE THIS AS A LEADER?	HOW COULD ASHA USE THIS AS A FOLLOWER?
Drives	Drive to learn	Encourage people to learn together and to share experiences. Develop goals that will stretch the team.	Take on training. Look for opportunities to be stretched and learn outside her comfort zone.
Skills	Relating to people	Identify what people care about, where their strengths lie and use these proactively in project work.	Use her skills to network with other groups and then feed back ideas and concerns to managers.
Inclinations	Prefers the role of 'coordinator'	Delegate effectively to build a more capable team, putting time aside to support the people and the process.	Take on a planning role.
Power	People wish to please her	Create a fair and open reward system to motivate her team.	Be courteous, notice good work and thank people.

Can you see the connection between Asha's natural strengths and what she could do with them? Applying them will come easily to her *because* they are strengths. Can you also see how much more positively influential she will become in being a leader and a follower who helps the team to achieve and grow? Notice also that this effect is potentially multiplied by combining the strengths across the domains.

Could you construct such a table based on your own strengths? Although theoretical, it can help us to clarify our strengths and as we become increasingly aware of them, we can look for the opportunities to put them to use. Although it takes courage and effort to re-examine our strengths and combine them well, it is valuable, as this is where we are at our most helpful to our teams.

As we reach the end of this chapter, take a look again at the introduction to section two. As we strive to become our 'best selves', we can take what we have learned in this chapter and combine it with the insights we gained earlier about our integrity and authenticity. In so doing, the most positive influence that we can have as leaders will be born.

Over the stile

What we have considered can help us to be strong both at a personal level and through this, at a collective level. Good leaders take the trouble to encourage this within individuals. Great leaders go further and develop the team so that the strengths of individuals become complementary to each other.

It may seem that the best outcome would be for the team to be harmonious and for people to suppress their individuality in favour of the good of the majority. However, denying our individuality, our uniqueness, can be bad for our teams and for our future, and in the next chapter we will consider why it isn't wise to conform too much.

References

1. Rath, T. (2007). *Strengthsfinder 2.0 Tom Rath Pub.* New York: Gallup Press.
2. Dryden, W. (Editor). (1996). *Developments in Psychotherapy, Historical Perspectives.* London, UK: Sage Publications.
3. DTI Insight to action questionnaire. Available http://www.inspiredleadership.org.uk/welcome1.php. Accessed 19 January 2019.
4. Maslow, A.H. (1943). A theory of human motivation. *Psychological Review* 50(4), 370–396.
5. Pendleton, D. & Furnham, A. (2012). *Leadership: All You Need to Know.* Basingstoke, UK: Palgrave Macmillan. The Primary colours model is ®registered trademark of the Edgecumbe Consulting Group Ltd.
6. Meredith Belbin, R. (2010). *Team Roles at Work.* Routledge.
7. Goldberg, L.R. (1992). The development of markers for the Big-Five factor structure. *Psychological Assessment* 4(1), 26.
8. Raven, B.H. (2008). The bases of power and the power/interaction model of interpersonal influence. *Analyses of Social Issues and Public Policy* 8(1), 1–22.

6

Don't fit in

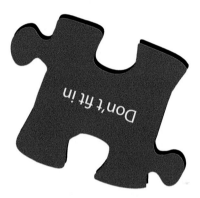

In this chapter, we will explore these questions:

- What does being unique mean and how does it help?
- How does our individuality help us to connect with the wider community?
- How can we balance being different with belonging: being me *and* being we?

Be yourself. Everyone else is already taken.

Oscar Wilde

Becoming uniquely valuable

This builds on the ideas that we discussed in Chapters 4 and 5 around being genuinely ourselves and using our strengths. Here we suggest that being ourselves is important to our collective diversity but, first, let's clarify something about the 'D' word. Diversity is not about political correctness, which can quite often seem like tokenism. Instead, we can think of diversity as being both a gift and a necessity because without it, it's hard to evolve and become better adapted. Why is that?

We differ, especially in our combination of strengths. Through that, between us we have different perspectives, more and better ideas and more and better ways of problem-solving. So, rather than get irritated by people who are not 'just like us', which is a commonplace and natural reaction, how could we cultivate what's useful about everyone's uniqueness for the benefit of us all?

It is worth reminding ourselves that strengths are not 'good' but are powerful attributes that are effective or less effective in helping us work together, depending on how and where they are applied. The combination of strengths is unique to each of us and just as with personality types, there is no rank order between them. The challenge is to transform what is uniquely *different* about each of us into something that is uniquely *valuable* about each of us.

On the face of it this notion feels comfortable, but because of personal biases and experience, it can be hard to feel neutral about people's characteristics. In particular, it can be hard not to frame some characteristics as being negative and our challenge, therefore, is not to let this stand in the way.

Case example

To give an example, suppose we had a colleague who was enthusiastic, optimistic and was amongst the first to put themselves forward for a new project. Trouble is that they could not be relied upon to carry through. Their strength did not lie in completion, but in getting things started through identifying the people and the resources that were needed. If we could recognise this, we could avoid getting irritated and disappointed by their lack of ability to complete the task, and instead, use their energy and networking skills to get new ideas off the ground.

Taking another aspect of being unique, through who and what we are, we may find ourselves representing people in our community whom we reflect in some way. This may be in obvious ways, like being from an ethnic minority, a particular religion (or none), being female, disabled, young and so on. However, what we represent may be less obvious such as being an introvert, having a chronic condition or being a carer. Who do you represent, or more tellingly, who or what do other people think you represent? In addition, we uniquely reflect what has shaped us.

Case example

Colin is from Scotland and grew up holidaying in the remote islands. The harsh environment is in his blood and he can seem distanced and tough. However, Colin uses this in his work. He admires and feels empathy for people who are marginalised and live tough lives and this has made him value 'fairness' and driven him to fight for the practice to address health inequalities.

All of these factors contribute to our differences and enrich the perspectives we have as a team and the quality of how we think and what we do. It's the antidote to being 'corporate' and becoming absorbed in groupthink, and can stimulate the practice to become more creative and adaptable.

Uniqueness, being our essence, has the power to encourage communities to move in a new direction, even though this may take time.

Case example

Deepak, a city lad, grew up loving nature and spending as much time as he could in the forests. In the 1980s, he became heartbroken about the damage he was seeing to the environment and changed his lifestyle and started encouraging others to take notice and change. For years, he was a lone voice in the practice – even a bit of a nuisance – and was characterised as a crank. However, people increasingly took notice and took steps to be greener and encourage this in the wider community. Even though Deepak wouldn't seek this, he is now seen as a pioneer and local hero.

We will revisit uniqueness in Chapter 14 when we consider its connection with motivation.

Being courageous and not fitting in to please people

Working with people or being in any form of meaningful relationship always benefits from accommodation and civility. Our social customs keep us rubbing along together and stop us going to war with each other. However, when it matters, for example where we feel there are risks in just going along with what's being suggested or risks in not speaking out, we may face a dilemma. This is particularly so when the team's core purpose and values are at risk. If these are being overlooked or sidelined, we may need to speak up for what we think is right and have the courage to resist the pressure to conform and to avoid rocking the boat.

Case example

Rachel was a junior receptionist working two days a week. The practice wanted the receptionists to support the nurses by taking on minor clinical duties but the older receptionists were set against this and tried to block the move. Rachel volunteered because it was what the practice and the patients needed and in doing so, faced accusations of disloyalty from her team. It was hard for her, but the practice supported her and she later went on to train as a health care assistant. However, her actions changed the receptionists' approach over time, and they became less obstructive to innovation.

We are not just ingredients in a recipe for the success of the practice. Our differences provide the heat without which nothing cooks. Being ourselves, being different, having the courage to speak out: these are all ways in which we can bring what's unique about us to the work we do together. However, the very act of doing this can highlight how we are different from the group and that can make us feel vulnerable and at risk of being marginalised or even disowned.

This reflects a tension at a deeper level between our human needs to be ourselves as independent individuals but also to feel a sense of belonging to the group that we care about. It's not easy, but our task as leaders is to allow, indeed encourage, both of these to co-exist. We can take the trouble to find out in what ways people are unique and create opportunities for them to use that. When we witness courage, we can recognise and applaud it, stand by the courageous and even protect them so that they do not feel marginalised. We can help uniqueness to be valued by the team, by showing how it makes us all stronger.

In these ways, a team in which people feel that they are valued enough by each other to speak up and be different, becomes a group with perhaps the greatest sense of belonging of all.

Over the stile

As we've seen, there is a constant tension between the attitudes and behaviours that help us to 'fit in' and avoid rocking the boat, and those that assert our individuality and the way in which we see the world differently from others. Both are needed if we are to evolve.

Part of our individuality is that there are boundaries that define us and make us unique. As we will see in the next chapter, these same boundaries are a form of 'limit' but interestingly, they need not be a limitation on development or influence if we learn to look at them in a different way.

7

Use your limits

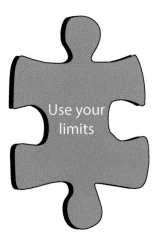

In this chapter, we will explore these questions:

- Aren't our limits there to be overcome?
- How can awareness of our limits show us if we are getting it right?
- Can't we limit our actions so that they don't cast a shadow on others?

This unusual way of thinking about our behaviour and abilities brings together some thoughts about limits and limitations including what we are capable of, how we under- and overplay ourselves and how our presence not only influences but also inadvertently limits others.

Seeing our limits as opportunities

In our everyday jobs we are used to the idea that we have limits, thank goodness, because it means we don't have to do it all. Our limits can of course show where we need to expand our boundaries by clarifying areas in which we need to grow. For example, all managers need to develop leadership skills and all leaders need to develop management skills. In this way, both can become more effective in their principal role.

However, because we need a team of people to provide health care, the limits we have as individuals create opportunities for others in the wider group, as we saw in Chapter 5 through the 'primary colours' of leadership. There, we also clarified that no effective leader is equally strong in all three colours, not because of any personal failing but because that is the way we are made.

Complete teams are made from

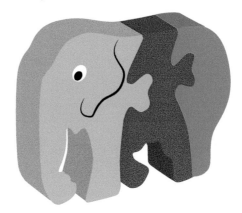

Incomplete people

Because the reality is that we can never be complete and therefore self-sufficient as individuals, using the word 'incomplete' is useful because it reminds us that we need others. It also stops us feeling guilty about what we lack and it modifies any arrogant or misplaced tendency to control people rather than collaborate with them.

Limits are also opportunities because they show us where we need to work around our deficiencies by bringing in people who are strong where we are not. We can therefore use our limits to grow others in the team. This also encourages our altruism so that we are less self-oriented. We can now see why it is important, rather than just interesting, to find out where the strengths lie amongst our team members. In so doing, we can build a 'complete' team where all the important skills that change requires are adequately represented.

At a human level, people who are strong where we are weak can be challenging because their differences and lack of common ground make them harder to connect with. For the same reason, they will probably find us difficult too. This can stand in the way of us being able to see each other's differences as a strength rather than as an annoyance. It can also impair our willingness to create opportunities for them, or to support them to make the most of their 'irritating' gift.

Look back at the example of Penny in the Belbin section of Chapter 5. Suppose that as a leader our natural inclination was to be agreeable and forgiving. Someone like Penny, with her capacity to push and thereby upset people, might be difficult for us to value, use and develop. However, good leadership requires us to do all three for the reasons that we have discussed. In the case of Penny, a good leader would help her to maintain her strength whilst encouraging her to develop her communication skills. Such a leader would also help her to value the differences in others.

Our limits are complementary

As shown by the elephant figure in the previous section, our limits don't just mark our boundaries but they indicate how we can re-shape ourselves to fit better with our colleagues so that we can collaborate more effectively. For example, shaping ourselves to preferences such as their wish to communicate face-to-face rather than by email, to use facts and figures rather than abstract ideas, to meet outside work rather than in an office and so on.

Case example

Steve has a strong imagination and is also a bit of a dreamer. He puts this to use in the team by thinking broadly and contributing to strategy. He always had difficulties with Li because she was not interested in ideas as such but came alive when putting ideas to action. They both found each other very irritating until they had a difficult but helpful conversation in which they opened up about how they felt about each other. This led them to communicate better and, later, to help each other to develop better ideas and more appropriate ways of implementing them. As a result, they moved from being annoyed and irritated with one another to respecting and supporting each other and becoming more effective.

This example also helps us to appreciate that we are strong in some areas *because* we are weaker in others. For example, big-picture people can't easily think broadly if they are obsessed with smaller details like practicalities and vice versa. We can also see that it is nonsensical (although human) to ask which is the more valuable member of the team. As the image shows, no part of the elephant has life or meaning without the rest of the body of abilities.

How our limits show us if we are getting it right

Our influence partly derives from our attributes and we employ each of these on a continuum from being underused to overused. Our 'limits' in this context are the limits on each continuum between which we usually operate. Through self-awareness and feedback, we can find where we are located and seek to be in the Goldilocks or 'just right' position.

We can appreciate this concept through considering five of our most important attributes (1).

MY ATTRIBUTES	IF I SHOW TOO LITTLE OF THIS I COME ACROSS AS	IF I SHOW ENOUGH OF THIS I COME ACROSS AS	IF I SHOW TOO MUCH OF THIS I COME ACROSS AS
Courage	Timid	Responsible/bold	Foolhardy
Integrity	Deceitful	Discreet/honest	Offensive
Flexibility	Obstinate	Persevering/flexible	Vacillating
Generosity	Severe	Encouraging/tolerant	Slack
Concern	Indifferent	Calm/warm	Manic

Here is an example based on 'integrity':

Case example

Hester likes to think of herself as a 'good' person and, although not pompous about it, she is open about her values and the importance of doing the right thing. Some colleagues feel that she overdoes this and signals her virtue too much. Because of her behaviour, they feel 'less good' than her, possibly even looked down upon, and this makes them feel angry and offended. The useful influence that Hester could have is being compromised by overplaying her integrity. How could we help her to get a better balance?

Have a look at the attributes in the table above and think about the feedback you get and what you've noticed about how people are with you.

Where do you get the balance 'just right' and where do you persistently over- or underplay yourself? It's interesting to note that personality has a part to play here. Extroversion accentuates the tendency to go to the right (too much) and introversion to the left (too little) in this table.

Casting a shadow: our behaviour has limits to the good it can do

As leaders, we can sometimes have a negative influence on our colleagues, but this is not always due to negative behaviours like the biases and prejudices that we discussed in Chapter 5. Sometimes, unconsciously, our well-intentioned behaviour or our personality will have limits of usefulness and can cast a shadow that prevents others from giving the best of themselves. The following table shows some examples.

OUR BEHAVIOUR	THE SHADOW THAT'S CAST AND WHAT A COLLEAGUE MIGHT FEEL
We are very hands on, into everything and possibly micro-managing our colleagues although with good intentions and with great personal effort.	The leader is doing everything and maybe doesn't have confidence that I will do it right. She clearly doesn't trust me, so why should I try to go the extra mile?
We are driven to succeed and use our ambition to be better than the competition.	The leader is very competitive. When he says it's about 'us', I don't believe it. It's about him and about being a winner and getting the credit. I don't want to be a competitor, so I'll just leave it to him to get on with it.
We have an extroverted personality and feel energised and stimulated through other people.	I know the leader is outgoing and enthusiastic and although this is good for the team, I feel drained by it and sometimes feel unable to cope. Because of this I find I can't be in her company for too long and what's worse is that I feel guilty about that too.
We are agreeable by nature and people find it easy to relate to us. We accept that disagreement and conflict happen, but we feel much happier when there is harmony.	I guess it's just the way I am, but I'm naturally critical and at times, suspicious of people and their motives. The leader is an easy-going person and likes people to get on. He is popular for this, but it makes it very hard for people like me to speak up. I feel marginalised because I don't think criticism is welcomed which is unfortunate, because I'm not trying to be negative but to point out difficult things that others seem to overlook or keep quiet about.

A good source to read more on this theme is Liz Wiseman, who in her book *Multipliers* (2) talks about how the behaviour of leaders can lead to them becoming 'accidental diminishers'.

So, what can we do to reduce our shadow? An overarching message is that we should be kind to ourselves and not get too concerned that whatever we do seems to have an adverse effect on somebody; that's life. In our efforts not to diminish others, we should not diminish ourselves. That doesn't of course excuse us from attending to behaviours that are seriously detrimental.

Opening up is key, and using the techniques discussed earlier helps us to appreciate how we are and how we come across. Our awareness of these techniques, especially in the moment, can help us to modify our behaviour in a way that helps others. For instance, we may tone down our extroverted behaviour and, instead of inviting an introverted colleague in a team meeting to speak, we may seek out their views in a quieter situation away from the crowd.

Over the stile

We've now completed our overview of the pieces of the leadership jigsaw that we highlighted. When working with people, we all have to learn the hard way, there isn't an opt-out from the inevitable knocks. However, what we have considered here will guide us, become more meaningful with time and will help us and especially our teams to have a better experience of working together. The insights that we gain here will help us to:

- Get a better sense of who we are and how to connect well with others,
- Spend our lives doing things that are meaningful and fulfilling, i.e., things that we *want* to do rather than just things we *can* do,
- Know what we are strong at, rather than just what we are capable of, and spend more time on these.

More importantly, understanding ourselves is a means to a greater end. By understanding the importance of purpose, values, diversity and behaviour, we can help others live more meaningful lives and move forward effectively and collectively.

Effective leaders help to develop great teams who, through communication and mutual respect, harness their differences in a common cause. How? Let's cross the stile to Section 3 to explore this further.

References

1. Davis, J. (2016). *The Greats on Leadership*, pp. 199–201. London, UK: Nicholas Brearley Publishing.
2. Wiseman, L. (2010). *Multipliers*. HarperCollins.

3

Our teams: Travelling well together

Section introduction

As leaders we are usually working to make improvements, but we can't do this in isolation. Leaders need followers and such people are much more engaged when they follow because they want to, rather than because they have to. So how can we encourage, rather than order people to follow us?

As we've explored in the previous chapters, it's about our influence and the key lesson is how we learn to appreciate what that is and how to use it better. The next stage of our journey focusses on how we apply the drives, strengths, skills and behaviours that constitute our influence and use these to get the best out of individuals and teams.

Most change happens when groups of people work collaboratively, not just alongside each other, over a period of time. Building effective teams can be one of the most important tasks we undertake as leaders. To achieve this, as a minimum we need to be good communicators with well-developed listening skills. This means listening with an open mind that permits thoughts and views to be changed by what we hear. Beyond this, we need to know how best to interact with people so that the team becomes greater than the sum of its parts.

As leaders, the work we do with people is often challenging and not always pleasant. Things don't always go well, and the performance and behaviour of others can sometimes work against the needs of our organisations, or adversely affect the rest of the team. Dealing with this can sometimes feel like walking a tightrope, and the choices we make about how we respond can sometimes have long term consequences for the culture of our workplace.

This section is therefore about how we build more effective relationships, in which influence is used well *with* individuals and *between* individuals, particularly in teams. We will explore how people connect with each other through communication and the art of relationship. We consider how to build capability through delegation, feedback and managing performance.

Beyond this, we discuss how teams form, grow and get the job done by developing mutual trust, motivation, mutual challenge and support. Finally, we consider how we survive and evolve through adaptability to both the expected and the unexpected.

8

How we communicate is a choice we make

In this chapter, we will explore these questions:

- Are good communication skills an innate part of who we are?
- Can we recognise and change the way we communicate with others to be more effective leaders?
- Can we be too empathic for our own good?

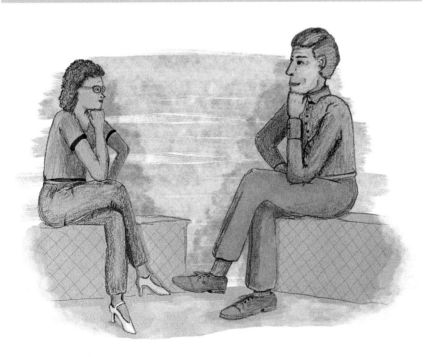

Good leadership is something that happens between people. Leading others is not something we do *to* them; it's more about how we influence their thoughts, feelings and behaviours by how we relate and interact with them. In every interaction with others we have choices to make, although more often we react based on our own values and the habits that we have embedded over years. How we respond has a significant impact on the outcome of the interaction. It takes practice to become aware there are choices to be made in any interaction. It takes even more practice to develop a new habit of choosing our responses wisely, and 'in the moment', with an understanding of the potential impact of the choice.

Our habits are part of who we are, and it can, at times, feel inauthentic to hold back on our 'natural' response to a situation. This chapter explores how we can develop more effective interactions with others whilst holding on to our authentic selves.

Why do we sometimes make bad communication choices?

In our imaginary practice, Dr A notices a pile of on-line shopping parcels that have appeared in the reception. They are all addressed to one of the receptionists. The receptionist is on duty at the time and so the GP chooses to say, 'Please don't get your parcels delivered to work, it's not appropriate and makes the place look so untidy'. Dr A then goes back to her consulting room, and doesn't give the issue another thought. Unfortunately, complex factors were at play.

DR A (PERSPECTIVE AND VALUES)	RECEPTIONIST (PERSPECTIVE AND VALUES)
Values tidiness	Doesn't notice mess
Feels embarrassed if visitors see the practice looking untidy	Believes that other people don't notice untidiness
Can't work effectively in a messy environment	Works well in a messy environment
Believes no-one can work effectively in a messy environment	Believes others work well in a messy environment
Tends to keep work and home life separate	Manages to work full-time as well as bring up a family but values a flexible working environment to be able to do this
Prefers people to give feedback straight away when needed rather than wait for a later time	Gets very embarrassed if she perceives she is being 'told off' in front of others; it reminds her of negative experiences she had at school

The impact of the interaction was confusion and embarrassment. The receptionist felt that Dr A undervalued her hard work, and she felt less motivated to take an active part in the project to improve practice efficiency.

What seems a simple interaction was actually a choice made by Dr A based on her own values and beliefs, with minimal understanding of the values and beliefs of her receptionist. It is easy to see why she may have made a different choice had she been more aware of the background and the potential impact.

Although it may not be possible for us to know everything we need to know to make an effective choice, being aware that our actions *are* choices is a good start. If we can optimise the way we that relate to others, we can increase our effectiveness as leaders.

Body language

Time and again researchers have shown that our non-verbal behaviour is more important than what we actually say when trying to communicate with others. In a well-known published study (Mehrabian and Ferris), 55% of communication is body language, 38% is the tone of voice, and 7% is the actual words spoken.

Our non-verbal behaviour is often habitual and automatic; it's something that we do without forethought, yet it has an impact on the outcome of an interaction. For instance, videos of GP or practice nurse consultations show us that if the clinician glances at the computer screen when the patient is about to reveal something of importance, the patient hesitates, and may not disclose. Similar body language used in relating to others in your team can have an impact on their contribution and therefore on your effectiveness as a leader.

Non-verbal behaviour is multi-faceted:

- Sitting or standing
- Eye contact
- Facial expression (smiling, frowning)
- Body posture
- Movements and gestures

Non-verbal behaviour can have both a positive and negative impact on communication and the impact is dependent on the meaning attributed to the observed behaviour by the observer. The attribution of meaning will depend on the observer's prior experiences and may relate to meaning drawn from different cultural backgrounds. Where there is a consistent attribution of meaning, there is more likely to be harmonious communication; discordant attribution of meaning can be problematic. Taking examples from the list above. If you decide to stay standing, whilst someone else is sitting, this could be perceived by one person as a way of asserting power, or by someone else as a signal that you don't have much time and need to convey the message quickly. For one person eye contact from the listener whilst they are speaking means they are being listened to and heard; for another person it may be interpreted as challenge. Many people find they naturally mirror the body posture of the person they are speaking to, something which is seen as a non-verbal way of expressing agreement or understanding.

An ability to read non-verbal communication can help us to understand why a conversation may not be achieving what we would like. Meetings are a good place to observe body language, and to consider what it might mean.

Activities to think about

The next time you are at a meeting, spend some time observing the body language and non-verbal actions of the people in the room, including the chair of the meeting. Does anyone put out their hand to 'stop' someone from speaking? Is anyone tapping on their phone or laptop? How do people demonstrate they are listening and engaged? If you get an opportunity to subtly observe a conversation between two people from a distance, check out the body language.

- Are they mirroring each other's body language? Check out for any avoidance of eye contact, crossed legs or folded arms. Do their facial expressions seem to reveal what they are feeling?
- What meaning could the receivers attribute to the body language?
- What might the impact be on the outcome of the conversation?

Social behaviour

Within an organisation there will be a wide variety of social behaviours, and each person will attribute different meaning to the behaviour of others. This may depend on their prior expectations. Social behaviours include how much time people spend sharing information about their weekend activities on a Monday morning, whether they share difficulties they are facing in their home life and whether they are prepared to be flexible in response to someone in need in the workplace.

If our social behaviours are discordant with the expectations of others, the impact can be a reduction in the sense of 'psychological safety' in an organisation. 'Psychological safety' is a shared belief across team members that they are safe to speak and act without fear of negative repercussions. We will expand on this concept further in the next chapter, but there are some key social behaviours that contribute to people feeling safe in their work environment. Something as simple as failing to return a smile from a colleague on arriving at work can have an impact on their day.

Case scenario

Jane was a ST3 in a practice. She was very sociable and used her social skills to build good relationships with the practice administrative staff. She quickly knew about their children, their hobbies and the ups and downs of their lives. That year she was given the task of arranging the practice Christmas celebration. In contrast to the previous year, the level of attendance at the celebration was high; following the event there was a significant change in how the staff embraced new projects, with a newfound enthusiasm for working together to solve problems.

Empathy

Empathy is defined differently by different researchers and psychologists, although generally it is considered to be the ability to sense the emotions of others and to be able to imagine what someone else may be thinking or feeling. Empathic resonance is when we feel the same emotion as the other person, in response to them. Doctors and nurses are taught to be empathic, but too much empathic resonance could lead to burn-out when they are dealing with people's pain and distress every day.

As leaders we need empathy skills to be able to 'read' a given situation/ interaction and to make more effective choices regarding what to say or do in response. We also need enough psychological distance so that we are able to be more objective in decisions and actions that are likely to affect some people more deeply and personally than others. Our ability to be empathic can be clouded by other influences, as well as factors related to our current personal circumstances and mental well-being.

Case scenario

Caroline is a practice manager at a small practice, with a list of 4500 patients, two practice nurses and one health care assistant. Janet, the health care assistant, started a period of sick leave to recover from surgery that was likely to be for 6 weeks, unfortunately at the start of the flu immunisation season. After one week of her absence, Tracey, one of the practice nurses, phoned up to say that she had fallen and broken her arm and was going to be in a plaster cast for 6 weeks. The nurse was a single parent with two young children.

Consider how important empathy is in choosing an appropriate response to Tracey's phone call. What could be the potential consequences to a response that lacked empathy?

Over the stile

By the time that we have reached adulthood, we will have developed many communication habits. Some of these will serve us well as leaders, and some less so. In the next chapter we explore the most important tools we have in communication – listening, speaking and the art of conversation.

9

The art of a good conversation

In this chapter, we will explore these questions:

- Is it possible to get better at conversations?
- How can better listening lead to better outcomes?
- How can we lead group conversations such that everyone feels heard?

Skill in effective dialogue or conversation is crucial to effective leadership. We know we have multiple conversations every day, and each conversation can feel very different, but we can't always work out why.

Some people feel if they are the 'leader', then they should be telling people what to do; a traditional view of a leader is that they are 'in control' and 'in the know'. However, leadership that is most likely to build a team and generate effective sustainable change relies on a different approach and is dependent on effective conversations with others.

Dialogue is something that happens between people, not something we do *to* others. Learning to have effective conversations is learning to gradually give up the effort of making others understand us, and learning how to develop a shared understanding. It is 'the art of thinking together'. We can process our thoughts more deeply when someone is actively listening to us.

There are two parts to dialogue: listening and speaking. Listening is an active process, not merely waiting for your turn to speak. Listening must influence what you say next. Real listening is allowing yourself to be changed by others. This takes courage and humility. As leaders, we sometimes feel we are expected to be the people with the right answers, so approaching a conversation with a genuinely open mind can be challenging.

Effective listening is an active process. Eliminating distractions will make it easier for us to spot verbal and non-verbal cues. One tip is to use open questions to try to understand the other person's perspective and then relax and stop talking. We can stop being frightened of silence. Silence usually signifies thinking and reflection.

Stephen Covey explores dialogue in his book *The Seven Habits of Highly Effective People*, with the habit 'Seek first to understand, then be understood'. An effective conversation requires us to listen empathically without colouring the contribution of others by our own view of the world. Covey tells us we usually listen 'autobiographically'; by this he means that we hear what is said through the cloud of our own experiences, beliefs and assumptions. Because of this we tend to respond in four ways:

We *evaluate*	We either agree or disagree
We *probe*	We ask questions from our own frame of reference
We *advise*	We suggest something based on our own experience
We *interpret*	We try to figure people out, their motives and behaviour, based on our own motives and behaviour

(Stephen Covey, 1st ed., 1992, p. 245)

John Heron, a pioneer in the field of participatory research methods, studied interactions between people, starting with GPs and their patients and then other interactions between people in a variety of work settings. He identified six styles on 'intervention' in a conversation, with each player having a personal preference based on personality, job role, upbringing, family norm and the expectations of others. We will be so well practised in our preferred style that it will have become a habit and we will forget that other response styles exist.

Push Styles

Prescribing	We draw on our own authority or expertise to give advice or direction.
Informing	Less authoritative than prescribing where knowledge and expertise are shared, without the expectation it will be acted on.
Challenging	We draw attention to the assumptions people may be making, to raise their awareness of the potential consequences of their actions or to draw attention to something we think may be happening 'off the radar' that others have not noticed.

(Continued)

Pull Styles

Discovering	We invite to others to open up about their thoughts.
Releasing	We help others to open up about their feelings.
Supporting	We build the confidence of others, reminding them of what is going well, encouraging further learning and taking of responsibility.

Most conversations, especially group conversations, such as those that take place at practice meetings, contain a mix of these preferences. Becoming more aware of these styles opens up the possibility of choosing different approaches when an alternative to our usual preference may be more appropriate.

There is a strong link between consultation skills that GPs learn through their training and some of the skills needed for having effective conversations in your practice. Understanding the ideas, concerns and expectations of the other person in the conversation will help you to shape and change your own views on the issues, and can lead to a shared understanding of the issue under discussion.

Case scenario

What follows are two versions of a conversation between Susan, a reception manager, and Tim, a GP partner. The GP also works for the local commissioning organisation and has been involved in designing a new local scheme related to improving GP access. The scheme has been launched and Susan has just had sight of it. She is concerned about how it will be received by the staff as it means spreading the working hours more evenly from 8am to 6.30pm and will prevent the practice from closing at lunchtime.

Version 1

Susan   *I've just seen the spec for the improving GP access scheme and I'm a bit worried.*

Tim   *There's nothing to be worried about, it's properly funded.*

Susan   *But I'm worried about whether I'll be able to persuade the reception staff to change their hours.*

Tim   *Well we can always change their contracts; how much notice do we need to give for a contract change?*

Susan	I'm not sure. And what about our lunchtime meeting – how are we going to all meet together if we can't lock the doors at lunchtime?
Tim	Couldn't there be a rota for staff to take it in turns to miss the meeting?
Susan	Yes, I suppose so. I don't think people are going to like it, though.
Tim	Can't you be a bit more positive about it? It took hours to design and I had to persuade two different committees, it was so much effort to get it properly funded.
Susan	Okay, sorry.

Version 2

Susan	I've just seen the spec for the improving GP access scheme and I'm a bit worried.
Tim	Okay, do you want to talk about it now?
Susan	That would be great, if you've got a few minutes.
Tim	Sure, so what are you thinking?
Susan	I'm thinking about the staff rotas partly, and I'm also worried about having to stay open at lunchtime on Wednesdays, when we have our full team meetings.
Tim	What's concerning you about the rotas?
Susan	Well, they are such a pain to organise and currently we work around the staff's childcare commitments.
Tim	Oh, I see. So it's going to take extra work to rearrange everything?
Susan	That's right.
Tim	I'm always pleased you put so much effort into helping the staff fit around their other commitments. It makes a big difference to morale.
Susan	Thanks. And I know they will try to be flexible if they can.
Tim	So what do you think will be the biggest challenges for cover?
Susan	I think the 5 to 6.30 times will be the hardest, as so many of the reception staff have young children.
Tim	There is some extra money attached to the scheme. If you were allowed to spend it on covering that time, what are your options?
Susan	Actually, it might be a good opportunity to get another apprentice. If we advertise the hours as including 5 to 6.30, then at least they will know in advance. We might even be able to get someone young who might be able to help us with some of the IT solutions the others struggle with.
Tim	That sounds like an idea worth pursuing. You also mentioned the lunchtime meetings.
Susan	Yes, I think everyone really values these, as it's really good for communication.
Tim	I agree, I'm always really proud that our practice still meets together so often, it helps us to 'get things done'.
Susan	Maybe we should ask the whole team if they can think of a way we could cover this, and still keep everyone 'in the loop'.
Tim	I agree, that sounds like a good way forward.

It isn't hard to see there are two completely different outcomes to these conversations, and yet the main difference was Tim's ability, in the second conversation, to put aside his own feelings about the scheme he had helped to design and instead to use genuine inquiry questions, actively listening to Susan to search for a win–win solution.

Sometimes we ask what we think is an inquiry question but get a reaction that we weren't expecting. This can happen if we fail to notice an implicit assumption embedded in the way that we have asked the question. In its simplest form, this is an assumption that the other person will know the answer. It's easiest to demonstrate this with an example.

> Tim asks Susan, 'When does the bid for the practice development money need to be submitted?' Susan may feel by what is seemingly a simple inquiry that Tim has assumed she knows the answer, but actually the bid wasn't something in which she had been involved. She may feel inadequate for not knowing the answer or she may even feel responsible for finding out, and then feel pressure, as she already has many tasks pending and this now feels like this is yet another one to add to the list.
>
> If Tim had asked, 'Do you know when the bid for the practice development money needs to be submitted', on hearing this question Susan would feel completely comfortable saying no, explaining that the practice manager is likely to know. She won't feel that she **should** have known the answer, nor would she feel responsible for finding out.

It takes practice to develop the awareness of our learned habits when asking questions. Some of us naturally ask one way, and some the other. People we work with will be aware they feel differently when asked almost the same thing by different people and may not be able to identify why. Learning to spot and remove our embedded assumptions can be so useful.

Group conversations

Group conversations are really important for teams to work together well. Leading this type of conversation is more complex than one-to-one interactions and can be fraught with difficulties. How comfortable people feel to express their thoughts and feelings in a group setting will be influenced by their past experience and on how safe they are feeling in the setting. Most members of a practice team will not have had training in effective dialogue or empathic listening and so can fall into repeated patterns of behaviour in meetings that can get in the way of the group exploring issues full, from all perspectives, before coming to a shared understanding of the problem and then generating ideas for a way forward. Those 'bad habits' can include individuals dominating the discussion due to strongly held opinions; lack of confidence to seek clarity of the issues due to not wanting to appear stupid; individuals who push for a decision/way forward quickly before the group have achieved a shared understanding of the problem; the 'quick thinkers' who can see a way forward and present this before others are ready to consider a solution, thereby missing the opportunity of a potentially better solution.

Suggested activity – How can we tell if we are leading effective group conversations?

Instead of thinking formulaically about the structure of group conversations, let's highlight five features of the way that people behave when together as a team, which are good indicators that the team is functioning well. Interestingly, each of these can be observed and measured:

- Everyone talks and listens to each other, roughly equally talking and listening. When they speak, they keep their contributions short to give each other space.
- People seem energised and, when they talk, they look at each other a lot rather than looking the other way.
- People don't seem to defer to the lead all the time but, instead, talk directly to each other.
- Within the team, people make connections with each other by carrying on side conversations in addition to the main business.
- People regularly go outside the group to find out more, explore and bring information back to share within the team.

Try looking for this within one of your practice teams. How does the team measure up?

Leading reflective group conversations

In Chapter 20, we share tools that can help us to have group conversations that encourage participation from all, whatever their natural style. Sometimes, however, it seems like too much work to do a full SWOT analysis or force field analysis when a group needs think about an experience and make a shared decision about something seemingly more minor. The ORID conversation method can provide a useful framework for this.

We are often too quick to evaluate our experiences and make sense of them as individuals, without incorporating how others experienced them into our conclusions. Emotional and intuitive responses are important, but we can dismiss them as being less important than that what we see as rational or logical responses. When we take emotional responses into consideration they can strengthen and support the decisions; if we ignore them we can jeopardise the decision.

The technique involves leading the group through four levels of questions:

1   Objective
2   Reflective
3   Interpretive
4   Decisional

Case scenario

You recently invited a representative from the Learning Disability (LD) Service to talk to the practice about how you can improve the care of patients with learning disability. The visitor brought data to show how the practice was falling short of local expectations in how many physical health checks had been done for this patient group. He asked what the practice was going to do to address these failings. He was met with an awkward silence. You felt embarrassed and morale was low at the practice for the rest of the week. You decide it might be useful to lead a conversation about the meeting. This prepares some questions to take the group through the four levels of reflection, as can be seen in the table.

Objective	• What did he say at the meeting? • What do you remember about the data? • What did we say in response? • What comments stood out?
Reflective	• What was the high point of the meeting? • What was the low point? • What were your feelings during the meeting? • How did we react as a group?

(Continued)

Case scenario (*Continued*)

Interpretive	• What was the most meaningful aspect of his presentation? • What was your key insight? • What can we conclude from the meeting? • What have we learned?
Decisional	• How, if at all, has the meeting changed your thinking? • What could we do differently, if anything?

The conversation took you by surprise. Allowing the group to think about what was said and how they felt during the experience helped them to recognise they had felt frustrated and underappreciated for the special care and attention they pay to people with LD. They felt that the key insight was that health checks on people with LD were 'business as usual' so hadn't been claiming a fee for them. Therefore, these checks had not been recorded, so it looked like they were delivering poor care.

Over the stile

Really good conversations are often the reason great things happen. This chapter has looked at some theory behind why some conversations seem more effective than others. In the next chapter, we explore team/group dynamics in more depth; however, the root of effective dynamics is often effective conversations in which people also notice and respond appropriately to the non-verbal signals that underpin the dialogue.

Bibliography

Covey, S.R. (2004). *The 7 Habits of Highly Effective People: Powerful Lessons in Personal Change*. London, UK: Simon & Schuster.

Heron, J. (1989). *Six Category Intervention*. Surrey, UK: University of Surrey.

Hogan, C. (2003). *Practical Facilitation: A Toolkit of Techniques*. London, UK: Kogan Page.

Issacs, W. (1999). *Dialogue and the Art of Thinking Together*. New York: Doubleday.

10

Navigating communication complexities

In this chapter, we will explore these questions:

- How can we work out what has gone wrong when communication fails?
- What does it mean to be assertive, and does it matter?
- Can we learn to use our power effectively and how can imbalances in power lead to communication difficulties?

Relationship dynamics

Really understanding the dynamics of a relationship between ourselves and others requires us first to have an awareness of ourselves and what we are bringing to the relationship. This includes how safe we feel in the environment, how we have experienced the issue we are talking about and the assumptions we make about the situation. However, all of this background is not necessarily known by us, or by the other party in the relationship. Johari's window, which we touched on in Chapter 4 in a different context, is a useful framework to use to understand this.

THE JOHARI WINDOW		
KNOWN TO OTHERS	OPEN KNOWN BY BOTH YOU AND OTHERS	BLIND SPOT UNKNOWN TO YOU BUT KNOWN BY OTHERS
UNKNOWN TO OTHERS	HIDDEN KNOWN TO YOU BUT NOT BY OTHERS	UNKNOWN UNKNOWN BY BOTH YOU AND OTHERS
	KNOWN BY YOU	UNKNOWN BY YOU

Each of the two people relating to each other bring their own sets of values, assumptions and experience that help to shape the relationship, and these are not necessarily known by either party. The more factors lying in our 'blind spot' or in the 'unknown' zones of this grid, the more opportunity there will be for miscommunications and ineffective conversations. As leaders, there are things we can do to expand the 'open' zone. Using Heron's 'Pull' style of conversation will reduce your blind spot, as it encourages the person you are speaking with to be more honest about their thoughts and feelings. Trusting people enough to start to disclose your own thoughts, including self-doubts, and allowing them the opportunity to explore this and to provide feedback can help open up the 'unknown zone' and help both to gain insight and build further trust.

Case scenario

Joan is a receptionist at a practice. She has worked there for 40 years and is close to retirement. The partners at the practice decided to give reception staff specific responsibilities around the practice. Dr C was asked to talk to Joan about her special responsibility, which was to be the maintenance of the waiting room space. At the end of the conversation Joan became tearful and said, 'I knew you all wanted me to retire'. Dr C had no idea what had triggered the response. How could Dr C uncover what was in his blind spot?

Our responses can have been shaped by our previous experiences as well as by our cultural beliefs and can vary widely. Our automatic responses could be considered our 'default setting'; if we understand these, we can better understand relationship dynamics and use this understanding to improve them if needed. An understanding of the theory of Transactional Analysis (TA) can help us to understand relationship dynamics, especially if there seem to be difficulties.

TA is a theory that originates in psychoanalysis and behavioural psychology and suggests that in any 'transaction' between two individuals, each party adopts one of three ego states: Adult, Parent or Child.

- We are operating in **Adult** mode when we are truly in the here and now, and not allowing our past thoughts, feelings and behaviours to interfere with our responses. This is clearly a very difficult thing to achieve and maintain.
- If we take on the **Parent** ego state, we use our experience of interactions with parents, teachers or carers from our past and channel these experiences into our responses. There are two sides to the parent ego state, the **Critical Parent** and the **Nurturing Parent**.
- In the **Child** ego state, we relive ways we thought and behaved as children, taking on one of two alternate states: the **Free Child** or the **Adaptive Child**.

Effective, positive interactions require each 'player' to remain in the Adult ego state. If we are spoken to by someone in the role of Parent, this can trigger a strong emotional response and encourages us to respond from our Child ego state.

Clues to ego states from language and behaviour

EGO STATE	CLUES
Critical (negative controlling) Parent	Frequent use of the words 'You should …' 'You must …' 'You never do what I ask …' 'Can everyone just stop what they are doing and listen …' Body language – finger pointing, hands on hips Voice raised
Nurturing (positive controlling) Parent	Gentle voice Warm empathic body language, concern for the well-being of others Tendency to want to put things right for others, even if it fosters dependency Delegation difficult as if the person being passed the task looks worried, the 'Parent' says 'it's fine, I'll do it'
Free Child	Expresses feelings rapidly and loudly Language uninhibited Creative and spontaneous Takes risks without awareness they are risks
Adaptive Child	Behaviours that are 'reactions' to others including 'digging their heels in', expressing anger, playing on mobile phone in meetings, using body language to express boredom, voice tone 'whingey' Alternatively: Overly compliant, agreeing with a request they may believe to be inappropriate but moaning about it later
Adult	Observant, seeks to understand the thoughts and feelings of others, can evaluate Voice tone even, with words chosen carefully

Individuals can move between ego states and are often triggered to do so by the ego state of the other person in the interaction. For example, an interaction with someone behaving as a Critical Parent often triggers the responder to take on an Adaptive Child ego state. Similarly, someone behaving as a Free Child can bring out the Critical Parent embedded within us, for example regarding risk-taking behaviour. Someone expressing sadness or fear in his or her Free Child State is likely to bring out our Nurturing Parent.

At times as a leader, it seems appropriate for us to take on the role of Nurturing Parent, especially if someone on the team has experienced upsetting news or has been badly affected by an adverse incident. Striving to choose responses that keep us in the Adult ego state will encourage others to respond in a similar way and generally creates more effective relationship dynamics.

Case scenario

Hailey is an apprentice receptionist. She has been working at the practice for three months and it is her first job. The other members of the administrative team are older than her, and grew up in an age before the rise of social media. The practice has no rules around the use of personal mobile phones at work, as they have never caused a problem. Hailey is used to having access to her phone all the time, and frequently checks her social media feeds, even during practice meetings and when she is on the phone to patients. One day Julie, the reception manager, can't take much more and shouts at her, saying, 'Are you tied to that phone? Can't you just get on with your work like everyone else?' Hailey immediately puts her phone away and goes quiet. Once Julie has left the reception area, she starts to moan about her behind her back, saying, 'Julie has always had it in for me', and for the next two weeks refuses to make eye contact with her, only responding to her requests with monosyllabic replies.

Which ego states were Julie and Hailey adopting? How could this interaction have been better handled?

Assertiveness

Assertiveness is our ability to express our thoughts and needs confidently and when we feel it is important to do so. Building on the TA theory described here, this generally requires us to be our Adult ego state. Often people are described as 'assertive' when they have strong opinions that are unshakeable that they try to force onto others. This is aggression, not assertiveness.

Leading others requires us to recognise the importance of assertiveness skills in the people we lead so they can safely share their thoughts and feelings, especially when things may not be going well for them. Effective, active listening encourages people to behave more assertively, as they feel safe to do so.

Assertiveness skills are particularly needed when having difficult conversations, or conversations with individuals who do not have well-developed listening skills. Being assertive requires us to be aware of our emotional responses to situations and to recognise and name our feelings.

Tips for assertive conversations

Be specific	Too much preamble or justification can dilute what we want to say and act as a distraction. Knowing that we have some uncomfortable issue to discuss can make us nervous, so it may be helpful to rehearse the opening phrases.
Own your feelings	Be prepared to share what we feel about something honestly, but don't blame this feeling on the behaviour of the other person. Don't say, 'You make me feel ...'. Take personal responsibility for our own feelings. 'When you said that the other day, I felt frustrated because ...' is more assertive.
Be prepared to handle the response	Needing to act assertively can be a result of a lack of listening skills in the person to whom we are speaking. This means that we need to be prepared for an initially negative response. This could include unjustified criticism or attempts to manipulate us. Stay calm. Seek clarity on the comments and listen out for underlying issues, including their motives and feelings. Make it clear what has been said has been heard, and summarise this back. If some of the criticism is just, accept and acknowledge this without becoming defensive, especially if it doesn't impact our argument.
Repeat your message	If the response does not address the issue that we brought up, then feel comfortable in repeating the message, several times if necessary. This is sometimes called the 'broken record technique'. We can continue to use the same prepared phrases, as this can help us to relax and not feel we have to think on our feet to avoid manipulation. This approach can be particularly useful if the person is aggressive and we are at risk of feeling bullied.
Aim for Win-Win	If we are actively listening, as well as being assertive, then we are likely to achieve a deeper understanding of the perspective of the other person, which may change our view on what outcome we were seeking. Being assertive does not mean always getting our own way, it just means ensuring we are heard. Seeking common ground and being prepared to cooperate and negotiate towards a situation about which we both feel happy where possible. It can be useful to think of the conversation not as 'you versus me' but as 'you and me versus the problem'.

Culture and assertiveness

How assertive we are is a result of our assumptions, values and beliefs, all of which have been determined by our prior experiences, including the cultural context of our lives so far. An awareness of the impact of context and culture on the levels of assertiveness in those we lead can help drive a deeper understanding of our team and encourage effective team behaviours. The GLOBE leadership study, published in 2004, assessed 62 different countries and identified some important cultural and leadership norms and differences in preferred communication style. The chart shown here summarises some of the findings.

Societies with Higher Assertiveness Tend to:	Societies with Low Assertiveness Tend to:
Have sympathy for the strong	Have sympathy for the weak
Believe anyone can succeed if they try hard enough	Associate competition with defeat and punishment
Value competition	Value cooperation
Value success and progress	Value people and warm relationships
Value direct communication	Speak indirectly and appreciate 'saving-face'
Have a 'just-world' belief	Have an 'unjust' world belief
Try to have control over their environment	Value harmony with their environment
Stress equity, competition and performance	Stress equality, solidarity and quality of life
Emphasize results over relationships	Emphasize tradition, seniority and experience
Build trust on the basis of capabilities	Think of others as inherently worthy of trust

The list is as applicable to individuals with different life experiences as it is to people from different countries. Understanding these cultural differences will help us to better interpret why different members of our team behave differently, especially if we lead a multi-cultural team of people from diverse backgrounds.

Understanding power

Our power is the extent to which we can control or influence the behaviour of others. Power is not something embedded within our DNA. It is not an innate trait of a person but, rather, something that is socially constructed by how we interpret what we see and hear of others as well as stories that we tell ourselves about our own abilities and influence. In Chapter 5 we discussed how an awareness of how people relate to us gives an indication of the sources of our power and how we might adapt to use our influence more effectively. Here we will discuss how power affects the way people relate to each other in a team.

Working well together requires recognition of power, and the source of power, particularly when we are interacting with people whom we perceive to have more power than we do. The dynamics of our relationships with people we perceive to have a different level of power or authority is often embedded in our past experience as well of the values we adopt as part of our upbringing and can be widely different across cultures.

Effective communication between ourselves and others in our team will be influenced by the relative feeling of power. Recognising where our power lies helps us to use it in a positive way. Practices where the power imbalances seem low (demonstrated by more informal relationships between the staff and the GPs, staff feeling comfortable to feedback concerns and issues) are said to have a 'flattened hierarchy'. This can help to generate a safe environment.

How comfortable we feel in a flattened hierarchy may relate to how this was managed in our home or school environment. Even in an organisation with a sense of a flattened hierarchy, the individuals will have very different feelings of power. As leaders we need to respect this, as an understanding of this will help to avoid unexpected difficulties in communication.

It can be useful to name and unpick some of the sources of power, both in ourselves and by thinking about how we perceive others. Note that this list isn't exhaustive.

Positional power	The power exerted by organisational hierarchy. The practice manager or GP is likely to be in a position of authority over other members of the team.
Reward	The power exerted by our ability to reward others, either financially or with praise and recognition.
Expert	The power exerted by our greater skill or expertise. This power imbalance is often present in doctor/patient communication.
Information	Knowledge is power. The more we know about a subject that others don't know, the more power we have. This applies equally to the number of people we know.
Referent/ Personal	The power exerted by good relationships with people, such that they comply with our wishes or agree with our approach based on loyalty and a desire to build or maintain a positive relationship. We work harder for people we like.
Coercive	The power exerted by our ability to make bad things happen for people if they don't do what we ask.

Case scenario

Angela is the ST3 GP Registrar at Kings Road Medical Centre. She started her post three weeks earlier and still feels a bit 'out of her depth' and reliant on the reception staff to guide her in many day-to-day issues. She is 10 years younger than the youngest member of the team.

One Monday morning she needs to make a referral to the Children's Community Nurses and goes into the reception area to ask how to do this. Jane, one of the receptionists, tells her the process, which is to print off a referral form, handwrite the details, phone it through to the referral line, and then the reception team faxes the completed form to the department. Angela declares, 'That's completely ridiculous' as she goes back into her room. Angela notices over the next few weeks that the reception staff start to treat her differently. They are less 'chatty' and start to refer to her as 'Dr Brown' rather than Angela. They are more deferential towards her. As a result she feels uncomfortable, and is cautious about asking for help when she isn't sure what to do.

We can analyse the dynamics of this situation, looking at sources of power.

POWER SOURCE	ANGELA	JANE
Position	As a doctor, Angela held positional power. However, as the newest member of the team, she failed to recognise this	Jane did not feel her position as receptionist was a source of power
Reward	Not applicable in this case study	Not applicable in this case study
Expert	Angela had worked elsewhere when referrals were all electronic so had the expertise of knowing the system could be better than it was	Jane did not design the different referral processes and has never been given the opportunity to influence them
Information	Angela is new to the practice and is not familiar with its processes	Jane held the information regarding the Community nurses

(Continued)

Case scenario (*Continued*)

POWER SOURCE	ANGELA	JANE
Referent/Personal	Angela had not been at the practice long enough for people to develop friendships or engender loyalty from others	The other receptionists witnessed Angela's outburst The receptionists feel very loyal to Jane
Coercive		Coercive power is often used at the practice to influence behaviour. Jane has been 'told off' before when she has made a mistake

Although Angela was expressing frustration with what she saw as bureaucratic process, this was interpreted by Jane and the other reception staff as an unfair 'telling off' because of the perceived power imbalances.

As power is a social construct, it can be deconstructed (or partially deconstructed) if the power imbalance is getting in the way of effective communication. You may not be able to escape from some aspects of positional power, but you can lessen the impact by meeting a team member in their space, or on neutral ground, rather than asking to speak to them in your office or consulting room. Being prepared to disclose areas of work where you feel less certain can create a better balance if you are perceived by others to be the 'expert in all things'.

Over the stile

The ability to communicate, both one-to-one and in a group situation, is the most important skill of an effective leader. Without this, it doesn't matter how many tools or techniques you know; people are unlikely to choose to follow you on your hike. We will never be perfect communicators, we will have ingrained habits that are hard to break, and we will always have an off day. This chapter has explored some of the elements of effective communication, as well as some of the pitfalls. In the next chapter, we explore how you use these communication skills to help people to grow and develop, not only to be part of your journey but also to develop their own.

Bibliography

Berne, E. (1964). *Games People Play: The Psychology of Human Relationships.* New York: Ballantine Books.

Heron, J. (1989). *Six Category Intervention.* Surrey, UK: University of Surrey.

House, R., Hanges, P.J., Javidan, M, Dorfman, P.W., & Gupta, V. (2004). *Culture, Leadership, and Organizations: The GLOBE Study of 62 Societies.* Thousand Oaks, CA: Sage Publications.

Wiggins, L., & Hunter, H. (2016). *Relational Change: The Art and Practice of Changing Organizations.* London, UK: Bloomsbury Business.

11

Help people to grow

In this chapter, we will explore these questions:

- Can leaders lead if they don't have any followers?
- Why is it so hard to delegate effectively, and how can we get this right?
- What are the different ways of helping others achieve their potential?

So far in this section, we have been delving into what it means to communicate effectively and how, as leaders we can build and work well with our teams. Our experience of talking to GPs and managers from various practices reveals that some feel frustrated with their team behaviour. They feel burdened with responsibility and would like their reception and administrative staff to take more initiative and participate more actively in projects to improve practice performance and patient experience. In this chapter, we will look at how, as leaders, we can encourage this in our teams by understanding what it means to be a follower and how we empower others by our own behaviour.

The importance of followers

Good leadership is something that happens between people, not something leaders impose on others. Leaders don't lead if no one follows. Leaders who impose their will on others will tend to create a very specific type of follower and may fail to recognise it is the skills and attributes of our followers that are crucial to the success, growth and happiness of our organisations. For decades, research into leadership focussed on the leader, although more recently business experts have been recognising the importance of *followership*. Understanding and nurturing our 'followers' will result in better long-term outcomes for our practice and patients, and will also result in a better-supported, more resilient leader.

Let's look at the impact of different types of 'followers' on what happens in our workplaces:

BEHAVIOUR	EXAMPLE
Do what they are told but don't use their initiative and are not particularly active participants	Staff who behave like this are often inflexible when faced with a problem, for example, at the front desk, that they have not encountered before resulting in a poor patient experience
'Yes-people' who always agree with the leader and will enthusiastically carry out tasks, but do not provide challenge	This team member may be good at implementing an idea you suggest and yet be so concerned to deliver that they may find ridiculous 'work arounds' when things don't go according to plan rather than let you know the idea isn't working
Deeply independent thinkers, who value this above committing to the leader; they may see themselves as 'mavericks' and can stifle progress with negativity	This person can suck the energy out of any meeting. If this is one of the doctors then, by the nature of their position, they can influence the culture of the organisation such that change feels impossible
Display some independent thinking and engagement, but can 'sit on the fence'	This kind of team member will encourage the maintenance of the 'status quo' rather than work towards change, if change risks disturbing their established working patterns

In no way do we suggest these roles and behaviours are fixed and can't be influenced. We believe we can influence our followers by looking at our own behaviour, particularly around delegation, empowerment and feedback.

Delegation and empowerment

Delegate: Entrust (a task or responsibility) to another person, typically one who is less senior than oneself.

Oxford English Dictionary

As leaders we are the people who are ultimately accountable for the performance of our practice and the quality of our patients' experience. However, although we are accountable, the delivery of care is shared with all of the people who work within the team. We entrust tasks to others by a process of delegation. Good delegation is an art; done well it empowers others and helps them develop their own skills, done badly it can frustrate our team and could lead to high staff turnover.

We delegate tasks constantly in general practice, tasks that have been 'part of the job' for years are delegated without much thought. For example, doctors delegate answering the phones, managing the appointment system and the repeat prescribing system to other people working in the team. Dealing with solicitors' requests and insurance companies usually happens in the background without GPs being aware of the process.

With many of these tasks we feel confident the staff can carry out their role without our interference because these were the roles they were employed and trained for and for many of these tasks we know they make a better job of it than we would. Delegation in these circumstances doesn't feel difficult at all.

It becomes more challenging when there is to be a change of direction, where a new responsibility has to be taken on, or when the outcome of the task is regarded as financially or reputationally critical. The internal struggle leaders have with delegating new roles or responsibilities can involve battling with our inner thoughts about ourselves, our team and the task itself.

Ourselves

We may feel guilty about 'dumping' jobs on other people that we feel we should be doing ourselves. This feeling may relate to how senior we feel and therefore how entitled we feel to ask others to perform tasks on our behalf.

We may feel, 'Do I have a right to ask someone to do this for me?' This could be particularly true for a new GP partner who may be younger that the rest of the staff, or a practice manager who has worked their way up through the ranks and previously felt of equal status to many of the staff. We can hold a fear of being perceived as demanding or inconsiderate of the needs of others and this could be especially true if we have been sensitised by being on the receiving end of poor or inappropriate delegation in the past.

Being accountable for the performance of others can feel a scary place to be and we might be tempted to assuage this anxiety by hanging on to tasks for the purpose of knowing that they have been carried out to the highest standards. This type of behaviour usually relates to new tasks, or things we feel we may do better than others. It is unlikely to be the case that a GP or practice manager would take over the answering of phones or booking appointments. Additionally, we may be fearful that asking for help with tasks could make us look weak or incompetent.

Sometimes we don't delegate effectively because we have a belief in our ability to carry out a task better than others. This belief will become self-fulfilling if we have never allowed others to grow or develop their skills.

Our team

Knowing how best to delegate, and who to delegate to, can uncover some gaps in our understanding of the existing roles and skills of our staff. We may be basing our decisions on a memory of a poorly delivered task in the past without knowing the reason for the performance on that occasion. Past experiences of poor delegation can render our staff fearful of agreeing to take on new things, and this fear makes us reticent about passing on new tasks.

Earlier in this chapter we presented Kelley's 'Types of Followers', and we could recognise some of these traits in the people with whom we have worked. The behaviour of followers influences how leaders behave, especially when it comes to delegation. It tempts us to only delegate to the 'conformist' or 'exemplary' followers risking over-burdening them and alienating the others. Repeatedly delegating tasks to the same people can soon become 'dumping'.

The task

We find some tasks much easier to delegate than others. The easiest are those where we believe someone else would do it better than we could. It becomes more difficult if it is a task we already do well, and efficiently, but have come to realise we have more complex work to do and need to pass on the responsibility to others. It is likely that when someone else first takes on the task, they may not do it to the same standard, and this will initially carry some risk that needs to be managed. The upfront time and effort it takes to support others to develop the skills and to manage the risk can be a significant barrier to delegating. The higher the risk, and the higher our perceived existing performance, the less likely we are to delegate, even if the benefits could be great.

The benefit of delegation

Good delegation releases time for the leaders of an organisation to direct their skills and resources to the tasks that only they can do. This may allow more time for the management of patients with complex needs, developing new services or becoming actively involved in wider networks of care across their locality. It can reduce stress levels in leaders and lead to a better work-life balance.

The world of front-line general practice is ever changing and needs to respond to changes in demand for services, altered needs and expectations of our patients and changes to technology. It's hard to keep up, but made unnecessarily harder if we don't make best use of all the resources we have at our disposal – most important, our human resources. Often the team members who are the closest to a problem come up with the best solutions if they feel they have permission to do so. Often 'giving permission' starts with good delegation. Delegation helps us to recognise and develop the talents and abilities of the team and generally results in greater efficiency as tasks can be done by the right person at the right time.

For many years, psychologists have researched the concept of 'locus of control'. The GPs and allied clinicians are used to considering this when consulting with patients who may benefit from a lifestyle change to improve their health. Our 'locus of control' is where we believe the control over our destiny lies, whether within our own hands or controlled by external factors, outwith our influence. If we have a strong internal locus of control and believe we can influence our own outcomes, this results in more active participation in managing, for example, our own health. If we have a strong external locus of control then we feel no power over our future and instead passively wait for things to happen to us, with no attempt to influence it. Many factors will have influenced the development of our 'locus of control' including childhood experiences and previous experiences in a work environment. In our workplace, team members with an external locus of control will struggle with the daily problem-solving needed at the front line of general practice. Lack of delegation can entrench an external locus of control as staff become conditioned to await instructions passively rather than develop their role or skills.

Delegation helps others to grow, and if done well, helps develop a sense of shared ownership over the running of the practice. Team members will feel more part of the wider organisational vision and objectives, which in turn improves staff retention and organisational resilience.

Looking for opportunities for delegation

Teams cannot function *without* tasks being delegated to them. This is why GPs don't usually answer phones or book appointments for patients as their skills are best used doing something else. However, we get entrenched in the established routines of who does what in the practice and we rarely take a step back to reassess. How wedded we are to our historic roles and responsibilities will be influenced by practice culture (we may value role continuity highly and see change as a threat) or it may be based on widely held assumptions about what the 'rules' are around who is qualified to perform certain tasks. Practices who welcome change and challenge myths can still be slow to spot opportunities for delegation because the area lies in their 'blind spot'. It can be useful to visit other practices to see what their habits are; they are unlikely to be the same as ours and helps us to realise there are very few 'rules' set by others, just habits we have developed over time.

There are opportunities everywhere, but we only spot them occasionally, often at times when workload rises such that we are forced to have a rethink. It is at times like this we need to proceed cautiously, being mindful that everyone is busy, and if the delegation is perceived as valuing one staff group (like the doctors) over another we may be setting ourselves up to fail. It can be viewed more positively if we look at roles and responsibilities proactively, for example, at appraisals or when there are staff changes.

How to get delegation right

The first step to good delegation is for us to be clear on the purpose (or purposes) of the delegation. Articulating this first can help us to avoid some of the pitfalls of poor delegation.

Let's look at some possible reasons we might want to delegate a task:

The task could be done by someone else, and if delegated, releases my time for other things that only I can do.

Sometimes we identify these tasks ourselves first, but sometimes other team members have been aware for some time that they could probably take on this task, but haven't felt able to say so as they were under the impression that this is how things had to be. A great example of this is the habit of GPs reading every item of incoming mail to the practice. It was only when this task became unachievable (with sometimes 50+ letters per GP per day) that this was questioned and the task started to be delegated. Articulating the purpose to those who will be taking it on can help them to feel enthusiastic about the change, especially if it leads to better care for patients, or easier access to appointments.

I enjoy doing this task, and am good at it. I am anxious it won't be done as well by someone else, but by hanging on to it I am preventing the development of the skills of my team and mean the practice is less resilient and flexible.

These tasks can be the hardest to pass on as giving up something we enjoy can be detrimental to our own job satisfaction. We may also have become entrenched in our belief that our way of doing it is the best way. This can stifle the creativity of others, who may approach the task differently. In these situations, depending on the task and risk involved, it can be helpful to delegate the outcome of what needs to be delivered and not exactly how to do it.

I want to delegate this task, as I really don't like doing it.

We all have parts of our job we don't enjoy, and we sometimes assume others won't enjoy them either; this can make us reticent about delegating. Sometimes delegating an unpleasant task can be perceived as a form of punishment. Being upfront about your own feelings about the task in advance of delegating can be helpful as you may be surprised to find someone is keen to help, either as they enjoy making life easier for others, or because they actually find the task interesting.

I want to delegate this task, as I don't know how to do it well.

This can be the most empowering form of delegation as it gives someone a free rein to be creative in their approach. It's an example of how we 'use our limits' as described in Chapter 7. It's important though, we remember, as leaders, we are still accountable for the outcome so need to be available to support and give feedback to whoever has taken on the task as they try out new things. An example of this kind of delegation would be allowing a reception manager to improve patient access to care by trying out different appointment booking processes.

Pitfalls in delegation

The three biggest pitfalls in delegation are:

1 *Time*

If you are giving someone a new task, what are they going to be able to stop doing to allow them time for it? It maybe they need to agree to more hours in their contract or that someone needs to be employed to take over some of the tasks they currently do. Sometimes delegation is an opportunity to take an overview of the tasks someone is being asked to do, to see if they are all still necessary. We can all be guilty of doing things 'because we have always done them' rather than because they add any value to either our organisation or our patients.

Do you have the time to explain the task? So often we don't delegate as it seems quicker to do it ourselves than to explain it to someone else and to handle the rework that might be needed in the early stages. If we are tempted to think like this, it can be useful to go back to basics and look at the overall benefits of delegation in the long term.

Be clear about the timescale for delivery, including the implications of it running over time.

2 *Skills*

We don't always know what skills there are in our team until we allow people to shine. In this situation it can be helpful to start small and build on what we already know the person is good at, and where their interests lie. Be prepared to be wrong. Even with enough support, some delegated tasks don't go as well as we might hope. Consider if the person could benefit from more training, or if someone else might be better at the task.

3 *Support*

Support is as much around our attitude as it is the time we need to allocate for support. If we are hoping someone will do a task exactly as we would have done, we are setting them up to fail. Make sure we are clear what is 'good enough' and be open-minded to new approaches, even if they don't quite achieve the standard of previous results at first. Would a failure be crucial? Or could it be viewed as 'nearly there and getting better'?

We need to make a clear distinction between support and micro-managing. It is better to clearly articulate the outcome desired, rather than the step-by-step approach, unless there really is only one way of achieving the outcome. When we first delegate tasks it is common for the person receiving the task to refer back to us if they hit a problem.

Whilst it is important for them to feel able to do this, how we respond can determine how they solve problems in the future. Asking for recommended solutions rather than stating what we would do will help them to develop their skills and confidence when tackling other new tasks. We will explore this later in the section on coaching.

Part of support is helping them understand the boundaries of their authority, meaning how far they are allowed to make decisions related to the task without referring to you. Are they being asked to come up with ideas for change, and then present them before implementing, or are they being asked to implement and feedback?

In Chapter 10 we used the lens of transactional analysis with its various ego states for Adult/Parent/Child to look at when communication within a workplace can go wrong. The success of our delegation is contingent on our ability to maintain adult-adult interactions with our team. Although, by the nature of being a leader in the organisation, we are likely to be in a position of authority over others, delegation is best dealt with as a meeting of collaborators, where each understands the needs of the other. The leader may desire more time to see complex patients, or to leave work on time, and engages the help and support of team members to look for ways of making this happen. In return the receptionist may long for the power to make simple changes to systems in order to be better able to meet the needs of patients who present at the front desk. In this way delegation can sometimes be seen as a form of 'trading', with each seeing what the other has to offer that may help them. As leaders aim to create the right environment for this kind of trading which can involve allowing all the permission to question usual habits and practices.

Creating zones of safe uncertainty

The concept of 'zones of safe uncertainty' is described in Wiggins and Hunter's book on Relational Change, and we feel it is useful when looking at how to empower a team through effective delegation. The best outcome of delegation is the development of a more creative team who feel they have both the power and skill to make a positive difference to our practice and our patients. This won't happen if the only tasks we delegate are those that could be achieved by following a simple 'step-by-step' cookbook-style approach. Delegating tasks where there is less certainty about how to achieve the endpoint needs an environment (or 'zone') to let this happen safely to encourage creativity, innovation and independence. This involves giving 'just enough' structure and 'just enough planning' and 'just enough' control to mitigate risks, but not so much to prevent people from wanting to try out new things and, if they don't work, to acknowledge they have failed, but feel happy they have learned from the experience. The 'just enough' structure could include ensuring time is allocated for conversations about the issue that is being addressed, but not requiring all these conversations to be minuted and reported upwards. Capturing 'next steps' on a whiteboard could be 'just enough' planning rather than the creation of a detailed project plan.

Creative problem-solving relies on a degree of 'not knowing', and this can make us feel vulnerable. We need to feel psychologically safe enough to stick our necks out without fear of losing our heads. A feeling of psychological safety is fragile and can be knocked by the slightest things; a colleague who doesn't acknowledge our greeting in the morning, a 'throw away' comment that belittles, having our ideas attributed to someone else or feeling blamed for something when it was due to circumstances beyond our control. None of us can behave 'perfectly' all of the time; we are all vulnerable to external distractions and stress, though it is useful to be aware of the importance of the small things that make others feel safe, or less safe.

Reward and feedback

In Chapter 3, we covered important aspects of human motivation theory, as well as how to apply this to encourage people to join you on your leadership hike. Getting the best out of others will always be easier once we have a good understanding of what motivates them and keeps them interested. This might be an intrinsic or an extrinsic motivating factor. In our experience it is rare for someone to work in a healthcare setting for just the salary at the end of the month. Most want to make a difference to others, or to the organisation, but we can sometimes take this for granted and forget to give positive feedback when we see this in action. Extra extrinsic rewards, such as financial incentives can be fraught with complexity, as those contributing to the achievement of something 'behind the scenes' may not be as recognised as those who speak openly about their achievements. However, simple rewards, like public or private recognition can go a long way to encourage positive behaviours and staff to continue to make suggestions and learn new skills. We discuss the broader context of motivation in Chapter 14.

Improving performance

Traditional general practices have generally not embraced the models of 'performance management' that are widely used in businesses outside healthcare or in larger healthcare organisations. These models involve individual team members setting their personal performance objectives for the year with their line manager and then being measured against these objectives as a way of determining if they have improved their performance. So, do we think general practice leaders have 'missed a trick' by not implementing formal performance management strategies? Not necessarily.

Improving a team member's performance is something leaders can influence with every interaction, and if this is 'saved up' for the annual performance meeting, or appraisal, hundreds of opportunities might be missed.

In 2002 Kahneman and Smith won the Nobel Prize for Economics for their work on integrating learning from psychology into economics, which became the origin of 'nudge theory'. Nudge theory is a way of understanding and influencing human thinking and behaviour to change behaviour by indirect encouragement and enablement. This academic work has dramatically affected thinking and methods for motivating and changing people, and runs contrary to traditional performance management and improvement models. Nudge theory advocates change in groups through indirect methods, rather than by direct enforcement or instruction.

The table below looks at the difference between more traditional performance management interventions and more modern 'nudge' interventions:

TRADITIONAL INTERVENTION	NUDGE INTERVENTION
Direct, obvious	Indirect, subtle
Judgemental	Non-judgemental
Deadlines	Open-ended
Persuasion, justify	Exposure to good role models
Limited options	Free choice
Paternalistic, parent-child	Adult-adult
Imposed action	Option of no action

Role modelling can act as a useful 'nudge' that influences the behaviour of others, and this can work both to improve and to the detriment of performance. A new member of the reception team can quickly lose their positive 'I'm here to help patients' attitude if they are constantly 'nudged' to behave differently by burned-out more experienced colleagues. A kitchen is more likely to be kept tidy if the cupboards are easy to access and the rubbish bins big enough to easily take the day's rubbish. Leading by using this principal means making it easier to do the right thing and more difficult to do the wrong thing.

As leaders we have an eye on performance, but if we recognise that the performance of individuals is heavily influenced by the environment in which they perform we have a better chance at choosing the right interventions for the outcomes we want.

Feedback and performance management

Positive feedback, used well, can be an important 'nudge' to embed good behaviours and performance in the teams we lead. It can be something as simple as noticing when a member of the reception team has handled a difficult query or a 'near-complaint' particularly well and as a result de-escalated a potentially challenging situation. Positive feedback is easy to give and lovely to receive. Some people feel greater reward if the positive feedback is given publicly, others prefer it to be given one-to-one.

Feedback about something we feel could have been managed better is more of a challenge but is something we get better at with practice. The first step is the listening, as with any effective communication. Stephen Covey says it well with his 'seek first to understand' habit from *The Seven Habits of Highly Effective People*. We can easily make assumptions about the action someone took, if we don't fully understand the circumstances or the thought processes of the person who decided to act in that way. It often turns out the persons choices were limited by circumstances we were unaware of.

For example, decisions made by reception staff about how to handle a specific patient query can vary widely (sometimes they might book the patient in for an appointment, or request for a GP or nurse to phone the patient, or send a query to an individual doctor). There is unlikely to be a 'perfect' way of responding to the query, so if the decision is contrary to what we think *should* have happened, start by separating the issue from the person. First have a conversation about the factors influencing the decision, which may mean the proposed feedback isn't needed at all, but that the issue has uncovered a problem with the practice processes such that patients and staff aren't sure how best to navigate them. Once you have listened, it may be clearer that the staff member was unaware that others approached the task differently and there is a preferred way. By depersonalising the event and trying to be objective, the team member has an opportunity to learn, without feeling chastised.

Being prepared to listen (in the true meaning of the word, not just waiting for our turn to speak) and explore the perspectives of others can be so helpful when giving negative feedback, for example, about issues such as behaviour in meetings or persistent lateness. If we truly value our staff as individuals, we will respect the fact they are human too, often with complex lives outside of work. Home life pressure and stress can spill over into working life and it is unreasonable to expect human beings to be able to separate the two all of the time. Understanding a little about what people are dealing with in their lives outside of work doesn't make negative feedback any easier to give, but it does make it less likely you need to give it, as you may come to understand the issue was a one-off, and related to a specific situation. Leaders who allow for some flexibility, as long as this is perceived to be fair by the rest of the team, will generally be rewarded by better performance in the long term. If the person with difficulties feels their leader tries to understand the issues, they are more likely to respond constructively to negative feedback.

Remember that what may feel like a very minor piece of informal negative feedback, may feel like a much bigger deal to the person receiving it. For this reason, it's still important to get the basics right.

- *Place* – make sure the conversation can't be overheard by others. Be mindful of the 'power' we might display by summoning someone to our room. If possible, find neutral territory. Being both sitting, or both standing can be useful.
- *Be specific* – mention the details of what the concern is about, avoid 'you always…'
- *Impact* – state the impact of the behaviour specifically. So for example, if they have arrived late for a meeting three weeks in a row, we might say that it makes us feel they don't think the meetings are important, and that we are concerned the decisions made at the meeting won't be implemented if they aren't aware of them.
- *Listen and learn* – find out what happened from their perspective with an open mind – be prepared to change our thinking.
- *Let them come up with a solution themselves,* if one is needed. They will value their solution far more than ours.
- *Next steps* – if the issue is one that has kept repeating itself, then agree some next steps.

Appraisals

Staff appraisal has been valued as an effective management process in general practice for years. If used well it gives an opportunity for dedicated time for individual team members to share their thoughts about their workplace and share ideas for their own, and the team development. If done badly, it can lead to a set of meaningless objectives and a strong sense of guilt year-on-year if these aren't 'achieved'. Remember that team skill development is more likely to relate to the circumstances that surround them and our ability to effectively encourage and delegate than it is to their annual objectives.

Pitfalls with appraisals

They are perceived by staff as performance management

Despite framing appraisals as an opportunity for a useful two-way conversation between a team member and a leader, they can continue to be perceived as performance management with a sense of 'passing' or 'failing'. This can act as a barrier to the type of conversation that can bring about useful change. Certain structural features of appraisal that we use year after year, such as formulaic pre-appraisal forms and the setting of targets or objectives can encourage and embed this view. If we feel these processes are not serving our organisations well, we can decide to do things completely differently. Remember, much of what we do is related to habits and myths about what we 'ought to do' that somehow make us feel more secure. That's not to say that encouraging some pre-appraisal reflection can't be useful, in fact it usually is. Just that each team member will reflect differently, and some will be stifled by having to write a coherent narrative about their achievements.

Saving up the feedback we have for our team until their appraisal is one sure way of making it feel like a performance management discussion. Feedback is best dealt with as close to the incident as possible, starting with listening to the circumstances. It's unlikely either we, or the team member, will remember the circumstances of individual incidents weeks after the event, which risks the discussion become more generalised, and thereby more threatening and less useful.

Team members can't see ways of developing their role

It can sometimes feel frustrating when members of the team seem unable to come up with ideas on how they would like to develop their role, or what skills they would like to build. This can be a feature of the arbitrary annual process. As we get better at delegation, the roles and skills will be developed gradually through the year and don't need to be 'saved up' for an annual discussion. If so, celebrate this as something positive.

However, it can also mean other things. It might mean our staffs aren't sure about the challenges facing the practice, or the overall vision or strategy and how they might contribute to the direction of travel. Appraisals are a perfect opportunity to share our thoughts and concerns about the future, and the challenges we see on the horizon and have a conversation about how they could help. Doing this well relies on us having a clear idea of ourselves of the overall practice strategy; without this our staff could leave feeling confused and anxious.

Sometimes team members are unaware of what opportunities might be available to them to develop new skills, or may be cautious about mentioning their desire to develop or change their role for fear this may mean they look like they aren't happy at work. In reality, we might also be unaware of the opportunities. Many general practices have successfully supported reception staff to become health care assistants, nursing assistants, managers and practice nurses using external sources of funding and apprenticeships. 'Growing our own' team using this approach goes a long way to making people feel valued, and results in effective succession planning.

Tips for useful appraisals

- Have a clear idea of the practice strategy and challenges likely to arise over the next few years
- Don't save up negative feedback for an annual appraisal discussion
- Use the opportunity to find out what they love most about their job
- Share what we like best about working with them
- Use the opportunity to strengthen relationships
- Seek feedback on how they feel the practice is performing, especially if there have been some recent changes
- Be humble and curious otherwise we will not hear what we most need to know
- Share the challenges and thoughts of the future in a way they can contribute
- Don't feel forced to create arbitrary annual objectives if this doesn't feel appropriate

Coaching and creating a coaching culture

Athletes have long used coaches as a way of improving their performance, but it is only in recent decades that this approach has been found to be useful in a business environment. In the world of sport, it became apparent that 'experts' in the field were not always the best coaches, as they tended to try to create replicas of themselves, and when this proved difficult, the individual being coached lost confidence and performance became worse rather than better. The best coaches seemed to be able to help the individual to connect with their innate abilities and generate self-awareness and confidence that achieved faster results. Imagine if we could apply this in our workplaces? Or get the benefit from it ourselves?

In general practice, we are more used to acting as mentors than coaches with our teams. Mentors have expertise and experience and use these to demonstrate how to perform a task or deliver a service to those new to the game. Mentorship can be very useful; mentors help a new team member to feel supported knowing they have someone to go to when confused by the complexity of health service systems and processes.

Coaching is a very different skill, and one that takes a bit of practice to get right. Coaches don't need to have any particular expertise in the area of work of the individual they are coaching; in fact, it can sometimes be detrimental if they do. Sometimes leadership can feel a lonely business, especially if we are starting to lead within an organisation that has fixed patterns of behaviour, with a hierarchy and a belief that the 'leader knows best'. Coaches can be a huge support for us, and help us to reflect on our behaviour and experiences to become more confident in our leadership and to try out new things. It's worth checking out what opportunities there are in your local area to connect with a coach.

As leaders, if we learn the principles of coaching, it can help us to get the best out of our own colleagues and teams. Applying these principles in feedback conversations, appraisals or situations when we are asked for advice can empower our teams and encourage them to problem-solve and think creatively, often generating solutions that go beyond how we may have approached the issue ourselves.

Thomas Crane (The Heart of Coaching) describes nine characteristics of what he calls the 'Transformational Coaching Process'.

It is based on data

A coaching conversation focusses on real events and the real feelings of the individual (*data*) and aims to be objective. It is hard for the coach to avoid making their own judgements and to park their opinions on what the individual *should* do or think, but crucial that they do so. This is when expertise can impair the coaching process and it is useful to be clear if the individual may just need some mentorship.

It is focussed on performance

The best coaching conversations take place when an individual wants something to be better but isn't entirely sure how to make this happen. This could relate to a practice system or process, a patient experience or one's own ability to carry out their role.

It is relationship focussed

Our effectiveness as coaches is dependent on the quality of our relationship with the individual. We need to trust in their ability to search for solutions and believe they are not just trying to pass on responsibility for something they are finding hard. They need to trust we aren't 'holding back the answers' in order to make them feel stupid, and that we believe in their potential to find solutions.

It is slower, not faster

In the constantly reactive, fast-paced work of front-line general practice it is tempting and at times essential to find quick answers. This can encourage us to develop the habit of offering our fast solution to queries, rather than to take the time to let someone think something through. If we get better at working out which issues genuinely need a fast answer, and those for which we can take more time, we will make better connections with people and help them to grow.

It requires more dialogue

Coaching is not based on telling. Good coaches assume nothing, ask questions, listen to answers, go deeper and explore options. This takes a mindset change for us as leaders, and it is easy to see why our own expertise can get in the way.

It requires more heart

Leaders who genuinely hold their teams in high regard, act with openness and compassion and are prepared to show their own vulnerability tend to generate better performance from their team. Bringing our 'hearts' to the workplace may not be something we have been conditioned to do. Some leaders have been conditioned to believe people will take advantage of them if they get too close to them. Interactions and behaviour is a two-way street. If we bring our hearts to work, others will too.

It requires humility

If we have a strongly held belief that we hold the answers, coaching conversations become difficult; as it is hard for this belief not to be transmitted by the way we ask questions or discuss options. We need to be genuinely open-minded, curious and prepared to be wrong about any assumptions we hold. The problem with assumptions, is that we are usually unaware they are assumptions unless we are prepared to let them be challenged.

It requires balance

The aim of a coaching conversation is to achieve a balance among thinking, feeling, and acting such that both performance and confidence improves.

It requires self-responsibility

If we are performing the role of a 'coach' we don't take responsibility for any actions that result from the conversation. This remains with the individual, who, through the conversation, has been given an opportunity to explore the impact of various options on both themselves and others. The approach encourages others to take conscious ownership of their thoughts, feelings, and behaviours and be accountable for the impact on others and the organisation.

There are both structured and unstructured opportunities for using a coaching approach in general practice. In our busy, often reactive world, the unstructured opportunities will present themselves more often, but we felt it could be useful to describe a structured approach, which could prove a useful alternative to use during appraisals.

Structured coaching conversations

Myles Downey described a useful model with the acronym TGROW in his book *Effective Coaching*. TGROW is presented here, with some examples of questions that a coach could ask:

1   Start by clarifying the topic for discussion (T – Topic)
    'What do you need to talk about today?'

2 Work out the purpose of the discussion (G – Goal)
   'What would you like to feel clearer about, or understand better by the end of the session today?'

3 Explore the current situation, including thoughts, feelings and behaviours (R – Reality)
   'Tell me about what happens at the moment for you?'

4 Identify potential changes or different approaches (O – Options)
   'What have you considered doing about it already?'

5 Decide what to do next, or what ideas to try out (W – Will/Wrap-up)
   'What do you want to try first? When?'

Some of these stages are easier for both coach and individual than others. Establishing the purpose of the discussion helps provide a clear focus, but it's easy to skirt over this in order to hear the details of the current dilemma.

The skill of the coach is to try to help the individual explore the current situation from perspectives they may not have considered and to follow verbal and non-verbal cues when these seem to indicate there are thoughts and feelings that haven't yet been articulated but might generate useful insights. If we use the sports coaching analogy, coaches and their athletes often watch back videos of the athlete's performance as a way of analysing and reflecting on the current performance. A coaching conversation can do the same. The coach helps their 'coachee' to reflect on real events and experiences, particularly the role they played in the event, as a way of analysing their performance.

The richer the conversation about the reality (and the reflection on current 'performance'), the more relevant the options for change. The more relevant the options, the more likely it is the individual will take something forward and try out something new, giving them an opportunity to improve performance, yet hanging on to ownership for the whole process.

Unfortunately, other than during staff appraisals, the time to have detailed coaching conversations with those we lead may seem a luxury we can't afford. However, the opportunity to have coaching-type brief conversations with our team occurs daily, and the main barrier to using the opportunity is our habits. The GPs and nurses amongst us have been particularly programmed to 'give advice' when asked, and this can be a hard habit to break. It's worth listening to the words we use when people come to us for help. Phrases like 'what I would do is …', 'what you need to do is …' and 'why don't you …' are often missed opportunities for taking a more coaching approach.

The difference in end result is best demonstrated with an example. In the scenario below, Jo, the reception manager has realised there is a problem with the staff rota such that there are fewer staff on the rota for Friday afternoons than any other afternoon. The Friday staff have complained they feel under pressure at this time, and feel the rota is unfair to them. Jo comes to see Sameena, the practice manager, for some advice on how to handle the situation.

Version 1

Jo   *Hi Sameena, have you got a few minutes to talk about the staff rota? I'm struggling to get keep everybody happy.*

Sameena *Sure. I know it's really difficult. There's always someone who isn't happy. What's the issue?*

Jo   *Well, there are only three admin staff who can work on a Friday afternoon, and on the other days we have four on duty in the afternoon. The three that work on Fridays say it can get really busy and they think it's unfair.*

Sameena *I remember this was brought up when I used to do the rotas. There's not much you can do without forcing one of the others to change their hours. Have you thought about asking them to do it in turns?*

Jo   *I supposed I could ask. What should I do if they say no?*

Sameena *Well then you might just need to be a bit more persuasive. Is there anything else I can help you with?*

Version 2

Jo   *Hi Sameena, have you got a few minutes to talk about the staff rota? I'm struggling to get keep everybody happy.*

Sameena *Sure. So what is it about the rotas you need to talk about?*

Jo   *Well, there are only three admin staff who can work on a Friday afternoon, and on the other days we have four on duty in the afternoon. The three that work on Fridays say it can get really busy and they think it's unfair.*

Sameena *Okay, so tell me what you'd like our chat to focus on – how can I be helpful?*

Jo   *I want to work out if there is a way to help the people who work on Friday afternoons to not feel 'hard done to'.*

Sameena *So tell me what you are thinking about Fridays.*

Jo   *Well, I have done a bit of analysis about workload on Fridays and actually there are fewer incoming calls, queries and prescriptions requests on Friday afternoons, so three people should be enough.*

Sameena *So it sounds like you don't think it's necessary to change the rota.*

Jo	*No, I don't. But I really don't want anyone to feel things are unfair. We usually have such a happy team.*
Sameena	*Tell me more about what they are feeling?*
Jo	*They seem to get anxious about getting all the tasks done before the weekend, especially dealing with the incoming mail.*
Sameena	*So it sounds like they are a pretty conscientious team. Is there anything that could happen to make them feel less anxious?*
Jo	*I guess if they realise I don't expect all non-urgent tasks to be cleared before the weekend, that might help.*
Sameena	*Anything else?*
Jo	*Thinking about it, the non-urgent mail could actually wait until Monday when we have more staff in.*
Sameena	*So you are wondering if taking one of the tasks off them on a Friday afternoon might make them feel less anxious.*
Jo	*Yes, that could really help. At least it's worth me talking to them about it to see what they think. Thanks for your help, Sameena.*

In the second version of the conversation, Sameena managed to suppress her own thoughts and experience about rota challenges and instead used questions that helped Jo to identify what she was really thinking about the dilemma, helping her to generate her own solutions.

Sometimes a coaching conversation isn't appropriate. Remember we do sometimes have useful experience or knowledge to impart, and it is perfectly fine to act as a mentor if the circumstances call for this. However, practicing a coaching approach can open up new solutions that are outwith our experience. It does take more time, but in the long term is a better way of empowering others and creating more leaders.

Some organisations now talk of 'generating a coaching culture' to create high-performance teams. The 'culture' of an organisation is the values, assumptions and behaviours that have become the norm for people who work there. It is often deeply embedded and hard to change. An organisation with a coaching culture is one that is 'feedback-rich' taking time to develop and maintain the quality of internal communications. Individuals welcome feedback and become used to coaching conversations as an effective way of developing their skills. Feedback isn't 'saved up' for annual appraisals and there is an on-going willingness to learn. A genuine coaching culture means the feedback is free-flowing in both directions, both from leader to team, and team to leader. This gives us real food for thought as leaders. Are we ready for our staff or colleagues to let us know the truth of how our behaviour is affecting them and the practice performance? Are we prepared to be coached, as well as to coach?

Over the stile

Helping others to reach their full potential so often requires us to stand back and give permission. To be authentic in this we need to become comfortable with things going in a direction we didn't expect or plan for. It means celebrating when others achieve things that we never thought possible, but it also means being prepared to accept people make mistakes, just as we do. In the next chapter, we explore one of the most challenging areas for many leaders – how to address performance problems and keep people in track.

Bibliography

Downey, M. (2003). *Effective Coaching* (3rd ed.). Texere Publishing.

Kelley, R. (1992). *The Power of Followership*. Bantam Dell.

Rotter, J.B. (1966). Generalized expectancies for internal versus external control of reinforcement. *Psychological Monographs: General and Applied* 80, 1–28. doi:10.1037/h0092976.

Wiggins, L. & Hunter, H. (2016). *Relational Change: The Art and Practice of Changing Organizations*. Bloomsbury Business.

12

Keep people on track

- Why do people get things wrong sometimes?
- What can we do to make things right?
- How can we prevent bad behaviour in the first place?

Diagnosing performance problems

If we think back to the last time that we took an exam, or produced a piece of work to a deadline, how well we performed was influenced by three key factors:

1 *Ability*

How capable we were to carry out the task. This might include the quality of the training we received, or it might have to do with our natural aptitude for the task.

2 *Motivation*

How much effort we put into it, which depends on how much we value the outcome, or what difference we felt it would make if we succeeded. If we are producing the work for someone else, our motivation will vary according to how much we care about the needs of the other person or the organisation and how valued we feel.

3   *Circumstances*

What things were distracting us, or making it more difficult to achieve what we hoped for. This can include whether we had the right resources around us to complete the task.

As leaders, if we notice problems relate to the performance of individuals in our team, it is useful to apply this thinking when trying to work out the best solution for the issue – first do your diagnosis. Getting this bit right is going to depend not only on us entering the discussion with few assumptions, but also on how comfortable (or safe) the individual feels to be honest. Finding a solution that works for both the individual and the organisation (a 'win-win') is ideal, though not always fully achievable. If both are open-minded and the space is 'safe', more creative solutions appear.

Formal performance management

When it does become necessary to give more formal negative feedback, we then enter the realm of performance management. Working out when an issue should be managed formally rather than informally is an art, rather than a science, and a decision that is best made by more than one person. Many practices get this wrong, sometimes by not knowing the formal processes or even by failing to follow their own procedures, leaving the practice vulnerable to legal redress and tribunals. No one expects us to be experts in this field, so get some advice from someone who is (for example a human resources company or the BMA) as early as possible.

In small organisations the impact of a staff member having formal performance management, or being taken down a disciplinary route, can be wide reaching and generate changes to team behaviour that can be long-lasting. Most organisations have (or should have) a formal disciplinary policy that was shared with staff at the time of their appointment, or following revisions. Being at risk of losing a job is a serious business so it is crucial that leaders take it seriously.

Consider formal performance management when there is repeated poor performance or behaviour that is having a negative impact on patient care or team morale, especially if there has been little change despite informal feedback. However, be aware of the potential impact of the decision.

FORMAL PERFORMANCE MANAGEMENT	AVOIDING FORMAL PERFORMANCE MANAGEMENT
The rest of the team may become fearful that their behaviour is being scrutinised, and feel less able to trust the leaders.	The rest of the team may feel let down by the leaders, and feel they don't care about poor behaviour of their colleague.
Time-consuming, requires careful documentation, usually there are 'stages' required by policy. During the process the performance of the individual can get worse (although it may improve).	The behaviour continues, risking the reputation of the practice and impacting patient care.
The member of staff may resign to avoid the process, which could mean a lost opportunity to help them improve their performance or change their behaviour.	Missed opportunity to eventually dismiss a team member who may be having a detrimental effect on practice culture and team morale.
Risks legal challenge if procedures are not properly followed.	

As leaders and/or employers involved in performance management, we have a duty to respect the confidentiality of the person involved. This almost inevitably leads to gossip and misinformation, with the staff member being fully able to share their side of the story with colleagues, who will only hear one side. This is less of a problem if the behaviour involved has been witnessed by all, but it can lead to confusion in an otherwise close-knit team who may struggle to understand what is happening.

Fortunately, in organisations with good communication and engagement, formal performance management processes are rarely needed.

Receiving difficult feedback

As leaders we learn how to give feedback and encourage others to develop their skills and improve their performance. We can practice the key skill of learning first to listen without prejudice, and reflect back what we may have witnessed, and to create a mutually agreeable way forwards. But what about when it is our turn to be on the receiving end of constructive criticism?

If as leaders, we find ourselves in this position, we could celebrate it. This may seem an odd thing to say, but the very nature of our positional power in organisations means leaders are very rarely on the receiving end of feedback. If we are, then we must have done something right to enable a peer or member of our team to feel able to let us know something about our impact on others. Remembering this can make it easier to welcome the feedback, even if we aren't sure we agree with it.

One of the great challenges to us developing our own leadership skills are our blind spots. The things people know about our behaviour and its impact that we fail to recognise. This can be particularly true when considering the 'shadow' of an over-played strength. If we are particularly strong in an area, for example 'seeing the bigger picture' and often present this at meetings, then this may confuse people with so much complexity they struggle to see what the next steps might be to any practice development.

If any of our interactions or behaviours has a negative impact, even if this was unintended and unpredictable, then it is far more dangerous not to know, than to know. But it is so difficult for people to tell us, and we will make this more difficult in the future if we react badly. If we handle it well and use it as an opportunity to learn and grow, then we will also have role-modelled the behaviour we want to encourage in others.

It's unrealistic to expect the feedback to always be delivered as carefully as we would like. Sometimes all we might get is a hint or a throwaway comment and it is very tempting to let these 'go over our heads' and miss the opportunity to explore the comment further for the sake of protecting our own feelings. Worse still we ruminate on the comment, with the potential to misinterpret what was meant or blow the issue up into something bigger.

Tips for receiving difficult feedback

1 Welcome it genuinely; as a leader you will rarely receive it.

2 Seek it out. If you get a hint, or hear a 'throwaway comment', find an opportunity to ask more.

3 Suppress any gut reaction to be defensive.

4 Ask questions about the impact of your behaviour on the feelings and behaviour of others.

5 Take some 'time out' to think about it, or to discuss it with someone you trust.

6 Arrange to follow it up later. Given a bit of time, you will have a new perspective on the issue, and so will the feedback giver.

Managing mischief and conflict

We are never our 'best selves' all of the time. This stands for us, as well as the people we work with and who work for us. Awkward or difficult behaviour (or 'mischief') can reverberate around an organisation, especially a small practice, and impact on how happy others feel at work. If left unchecked, this behaviour can become embedded into the culture of the organisation.

As leaders we aren't always around when the behaviour is being demonstrated, but we might pick it up via gossip, or by a sense of unease amongst other members of the team. Those who are exposed to it are likely to have their own assumptions, beliefs and opinions on the reasons for the behaviour, but be mindful that their interpretation may not be a true, or a complete picture.

If someone is feeling aggrieved or unhappy at work, they can feel isolated, and respond by trying to pull others with them on their journey of misery so that they feel less alone. If others disagree, it is easy to see how cliques and factions form. As leaders we might encourage this by 'siding' with those who are happy at work as this is where we feel most comfortable. This is likely to generate more polarisation.

From time to time, most organisations suffer from difficult relationships between team members, which can, at times, have a huge impact on everyone's happiness at work. Subtle negative behaviour can feel like bullying to someone feeling vulnerable and if persistent and left unchecked can result in loss of staff, formal bullying procedures and a demotivated team.

There will be underlying reasons for difficult relationships between staff, often related to differences in background, values and perceived levels of competence or laziness.

Every situation is likely to be unique, as it reflects the complexity of human feelings and behaviours but there are some basic principles that can be useful to keep in mind:

1   *Decide if it needs to be dealt with*
    The crucial first step is sometimes we need to pick our battles for the sake of our own well-being. However, don't ignore anything that seems to have been going on for more than a few weeks, and seems to be affecting staff morale. If difficult behaviour becomes embedded in culture, this is going to be really hard to set right.

2   *Don't just think about it alone*
    It is too easy to become wedded to our assumptions about causes and impact of behaviour. Other leaders within the practice that we trust may have useful insights and thoughts on background, impact and how the behaviour could be approached.

3 *Don't gossip*

   Although we may achieve a greater understanding of the behaviour by talking to others, restrict this to a few trusted people and frame the discussion about how to approach the behaviour, rather than encouraging lots of discussion behind the back of the person or people concerned.

4 *Check who is the right person to deal with it*

   This might not be us. If there is a line management structure in place, and the line manager has the right skills, then let them do their job. As these situations may not arise that often, it is possible that a reception manager has never had to deal with this type of thing before, so don't delegate and then leave them unsupported. Consider 'coaching' them through it.

5 *Assume there is a back-story, but don't assume what it is*

   Most 'mischief' occurs for a reason, and this could be complicated and involve things that have been happening at home as much as at work. If we assume there is a reason, but not what this is, we can be genuinely curious and are more likely to choose the right intervention.

6 *Be clear about what has been noticed and why it is a concern*

   When it comes to behaviours, there are rarely any absolute facts. If someone reports to us that they heard someone else saying something of concern, the person reporting the issue will have interpreted what they heard depending on their own assumptions about the meaning, and this will have influenced their report. The 'meaning' is an assumption, but the impact on how they felt when they heard it (or how we feel when we hear about it) is valid. When approaching a conversation about it, always bear this in mind.

7 *Remember the principles of effective dialogue*

   This includes the importance of inquiry and active listening. It's useful to hold an awareness of the power we hold and how this could impact the effectiveness of the conversation. Pick up on cues that may tell you the issue is deeper than first thought and know when to stop the conversation, and come back to it later if necessary.

8 *Don't fight back*

   We might be met with an aggressive defence response. It's never helpful to rise to this. Remember we are trying to neutralise the behaviour, not escalate it.

9   *Know the boundaries and be honest*

If, despite our best efforts, the behaviour and its impact on others goes unacknowledged than don't back away if we feel it is impacting team morale or performance. Formal performance management is an option. It's worth revisiting the conversation after a few days, as the initial response may be a defence mechanism that softens after time and reflection.

Preventing conflict and bad behaviour

It's unrealistic to think we can completely prevent bad behaviour all of the time, but we can lessen the likelihood of it occurring. So much of what we have been exploring so far in this book will go a long way to helping our practices to be happy places to work. If we act as good role models, including being prepared to take feedback and learn from our own mistakes we will help others to be less defensive. If people feel heard, and are given the opportunity to express their concerns, there is less need for bad behaviour.

On many occasions conflict between people at work can occur if the people come from such different backgrounds they are perceived as 'other' and therefore, some kind of threat to identity. There can also be conflict related to how efficient or effective (or 'lazy') people within teams are perceived by others. For example, a GP who is really good at communicating with people may not be as good at delivering on promises to update protocols or manage finances. This can generate conflict between GP partners. If we are genuine in how we welcome diversity of background, opinion and strengths then people will feel valued for their unique perspective. Demonstrating this can help others in our team to celebrate differences and minimise conflict.

At times people behave badly because they feel they have been treated badly. As far as it is in our power, we can ensure that people are remunerated fairly, have enough time in their working hours to achieve what they are asked to do, and have the right resources to get the job done.

Remembering that leading is about relating to people. If people see us as unique human beings, and we see them in this way too, bad behaviour decreases. This means there *is* value to conversations about our lives outside of work. These help to build a sense of who we are as people so that we all get better at understanding each other.

Over the stile

We have learnt much about how we apply our understanding of ourselves in order to understand others better. People's behaviour varies and we have considered how we avoid making assumptions, learn about back stories and help individuals to grow, sometimes despite their behaviour rather than because of it. We now move onto new terrain in which we consider how groups of individuals become teams and our part, as leaders, in helping them to become the best they are capable of.

13

Become a team

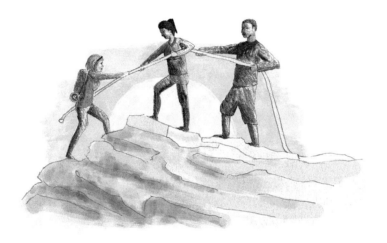

In this chapter, we will explore these questions:

- Do we need to be a team?
- Why is noticing people such a big deal?
- What are the four factors that all teams must address to be effective?
- Why do people need to bump into each other?
- How do we create an environment where people feel safe enough to trust each other?
- People rank themselves with respect to each other. Does this matter?

Introduction

In section two, we looked closely at our attributes as leaders and at a number of aspects of how people connect to each other and keep practice evolution on track. Because people are the building blocks of teams, how we think and behave as individuals become the building blocks of how we work together collectively.

We will now take the insights that we gained about ourselves and apply them to the group. We will consider how we move from being a collection of people to becoming a co-operative enterprise, which just to be clear, is not the same thing as a 'family' although it has some features (like commitment, passion and falling out) in common.

So, let's think about this group who work together. We commonly refer to them as our 'primary care team' but actually, are we a team? To find out, we can ask ourselves these questions (1):

- Do we have a clear task?
- Do we work closely together to achieve our objectives?
- Do we meet regularly to review performance and how it can be improved?

If we answer 'no' to one or more of these, it means we are not a team but something else. It's an interesting thought, because it can help us to appreciate why our primary care 'teams' might feel frustrated and perhaps let down. Although they are called a team, they may not have the clear focus, team leadership, regular meetings, and support that help real teams to be effective. So, rather than a team, it might be more helpful to think of them as a *community* that shares common values and the broad purpose of offering compassionate healthcare to our local population.

From this healthcare community, a number of real teams will arise. Some of them are stable and long-term, such as our practice nurse, managerial and reception teams. Others may be short-term, coming together to deliver a task by bringing in a range of people from across different groups to share their perspectives and skills.

So how does this realisation help us as leaders? First, it helps everyone to clarify expectations so that these appropriately reflect whether we are working in a real team or not.

Second, it helps us appreciate that when team-working is needed, we can facilitate this by attending to the people and to the task. This we do by improving the climate, particularly by helping people to relate better to the organisation and to each other. Aided by this climate, we can help create effective task-orientated groups, which are small and usually fewer than ten people.

Do we need a team?

Rather than make assumptions, we should recognise that tasks don't always need teams, so we should feel comfortable in managing without them where this is appropriate.

Case example

Peter maintains the IT in the practice. His skills are invaluable and he often assists in matters ranging from getting people on-line when their smart cards play up, to fixing printers or designing macros for new computerised templates. His tasks can usually be completed using his expertise alone and he rarely has the need to collaborate with a wider IT team.

Unlike in this situation, teams are needed when the task requires a range of skills from people who are dependent on each other's contribution. One issue is that because of the independent nature of the work, people like Peter may lack the experience of working with others and find it that much harder when the need arises, so it can help for leaders to recognise this gap and be on the lookout for team-working opportunities for people like Peter, when these arise.

What do people need in order to give their best in a team?

The elements we discuss below seem like common sense, but importantly, they are also evidence-based (1). Helping the team to work well together isn't rocket science, but how do we know that we're providing what is needed?

The evidence suggests that there are four key factors which we will now describe as they sketch the bigger picture for this chapter.

Compassion: People, especially in healthcare which has some of the most motivated people in any community, have the expectation of doing meaningful work. In healthcare our values are strong, especially the importance of caring, and if people are to feel engaged then this caring nature has to be respected, encouraged and given suitable outlets. If it isn't, we and our patients will suffer. When health systems go wrong, we often see that this vital need has not had sufficient attention because it has been assumed rather than addressed.

Although compassion is noted as a core value in clinicians, it's there in *every* team role. For example, we see it in our receptionists who go the extra mile to get a 'squeeze-in' appointment for an elderly patient who has come down to surgery. We also see it in our cleaner who doesn't feel s/he is cleaning the treatment room so much as preventing patients from picking up infections that could be avoided. As leaders we can applaud and reinforce these behaviours and attitudes.

Just as we show compassion to patients, compassion should begin at home and each and every member of our team needs to feel that they matter enough to be treated with care. Adopting a useful *mindset* can help us to behave better with each other, for example, by thinking of our team members as friends or potential friends rather than just as employees or colleagues. This mindset encourages us to treat others with more respect, take interest in their lives and show compassion and support. It also reduces the status gap and allows those with lower status to offer advice and help more easily. A different imaginary relationship might work for you.

As leaders, modelling greater equality can help shape the behaviour of our colleagues, especially those with greater power. For example, in such a climate, it no longer becomes acceptable for more senior colleagues to fail to welcome newcomers.

Our primary purpose is to care for patients and the evidence is that our personal capacity to do this, is related, pretty directly to the interest and care we ourselves receive. Often, this won't be asked for, but if it is overlooked, we can end up not knowing each other well enough to notice when attention might be welcomed.

Case example

Arjun, a GP in the practice, knew that John, a young physio, was going to become a dad in a few months' time. He made a note in his diary to speak to John a few days beforehand, check out how things were going and how he was feeling about the big day. John was nervous and wouldn't have brought it up, but Arjun's action made him feel better and made him feel even more strongly that he was valued by the team and that he belonged.

We can see from this example how the small stuff is actually the big stuff. Being noticed when what's happening in our lives isn't being broadcast, shows us that the people around us really care. As colleagues, but particularly as leaders, showing interest in the team on a daily basis is invaluable. Such things as knowing what's going on in people's lives, congratulating them on birthdays, asking how they are when a child is ill or when they just don't look right; these are the things that form the most powerful bonds. It is therefore no surprise to discover that it is this behaviour more than any other, that correlates with how 'good' a leader is thought to be by the team.

As leaders we can raise the profile of compassion. For example, by creating outlets for it through charitable activity such as sponsorship and volunteering or by showing our community how our work has compassion at its core. For instance, we may share a patient's positive feedback on how they were cared for or we may highlight the work that social prescribers are doing to tackle loneliness and isolation in the elderly.

Let's go broader; positive emotion of which compassion is an important example, makes people thrive and we should use every opportunity, such as giving an appropriate amount of praise or recognition, to nurture this. The evidence is that when people feel good, they experience better health and they treat each other and their patients better. Positivity and well-being are therefore related. Looking at this another way, we can think of this as a safety issue. Treating people *badly* leads to harm to colleagues and through this, harm to patients. So, treating people well is not just good, it is necessary.

Engagement: People engage more and therefore give more, when they have work that is both meaningful to them and challenging enough to help them develop without becoming overstretched. To be meaningful, there needs to be a core purpose and set of values with which their work resonates; this is part of what we call the organisation's 'vision'. Such a vision, as we discuss in Chapter 17, is clear but it's also compelling, because it makes people feel they *want* to strive for it.

When people are reminded through the achievements of the group, how their work connects strongly to the vision, their morale and engagement remain buoyant. As leaders, we have a pivotal role in helping the team develop its vision and in being its standard-bearer, keeping this in view of everyone when it matters. This is vital, now more than ever, when the pace of work and the competing priorities make it difficult to remember our core purpose, let alone connect with it. Doing so need not be grand or difficult as, for example, people respond powerfully to narrative. Healthcare has compassion at its heart and sharing the small everyday stories of thoughtfulness and kindness can be amongst the most significant things that we do. It is these things that remind everyone of who we are as a community and what matters to us.

Our role is not just to achieve success for the tasks, but success for the people, which means helping individuals and reminding people that everyone has the potential to develop regardless of formal education. We can encourage this by setting challenging tasks that go beyond following a protocol and that require initiative. Provided the tasks are appropriately set and supported, these 'stretch' opportunities stimulate people rather than burden them.

Clarity: The goals of the team have to be *few* enough to be feasible and *clear* enough so that people know what is expected of them and where the boundaries of the task and of appropriate behaviour lie. If these are not clear, our teams can become confused, anxious, frustrated and less able to apply themselves with strength and confidence.

Effective leadership: There are several leaders in any team at any time, such as GP partners, practice managers and nursing leaders, and inconsistent leadership *between* them as well as poor leadership by any *one* of them, can undermine a team's effectiveness. Leaders are role models and it is our behaviour in embodying the vision and creating the climate of compassion, engagement and clarity, that inspires confidence and helps the team to succeed.

Task and people

Teamwork is all about these two important elements and it's the task that generally determines whether a team of people is needed.

What do effective teams look like?

These are small enough to be well-functioning groups where everyone is necessary, and a common mistake is to have too many people. This may result from a lack of discipline in deciding who is essential rather than just desirable, or perhaps from a well-meaning but misguided desire to be 'inclusive' and give opportunities to more people.

Effective teams will have clearly defined goals that motivate, and the team members will have characteristics such as those we describe later in this chapter. Looked at another way, in poorly-functioning teams, people may not trust each other, open up or feel easy together. This adversely affects performance because people who are not jointly connected are rarely jointly committed.

Who should we get?

We should recruit the right people for what the task requires. Although this sounds obvious, it isn't always the reality. Such people will have strengths in the areas required and be a small but diverse group with different perspectives and skills. More subtly, we should avoid modifying the task too much around what we think people are capable of. This is because teamwork is a great opportunity for the innovation, creativity and learning that increases the capability of our team members and our practice.

Relating well

People give their best when they feel encouraged to contribute and when their needs are met through their work. To make this possible, people have to relate well to each other, and we'll now explore what it takes to do that.

Bump in to each other

If people are going to work well together, they have to feel comfortable with, rather than suspicious of, each other. To achieve that, people need to meet or at least come across each other frequently enough. If this doesn't happen, relationships don't grow as people do not become familiar enough to start to trust and care about each other.

We may not notice in our practice, but people can become physically isolated. The GPs in their consulting rooms are a classic example and unless they come out of their private spaces, they may go for most of the day without interacting with other team members. The same happens when people work virtually or away, from the main site, maybe in a branch surgery or at home. Does that sound familiar?

Additionally, even when people are together in shared office space, they may not be conversing with each other. Take a look at open plan offices with hot-desks and glass walls. Although these might be thought to encourage communication, the opposite can happen if people feel they are in a goldfish bowl, being watched to make sure they are getting on with their work rather than talking to each other. However, talking (within limits of course) is not time wasted because if people aren't communicating and relating, then the practice isn't developing.

Making assumptions that people will start to become familiar with each other through the infrequent formal meetings that bring the group together, is probably a mistake. These situations are not relaxed environments and can be dangerous places to open up about ourselves with people we may not know well enough to trust without reservation.

Instead, people benefit from 'bumping-in' to each other by which we mean having unplanned, brief, repeated encounters where there are no 'agendas' and people feel sufficiently at ease to say hello and to share on a personal basis. Water coolers, coffee machines, seats around wherever we do our administrative work; these are all examples of how we can structure the workplace to make bumping-in inevitable. Unlike group meetings, these environments also suit introverts as well as extroverts.

It may not be practical for people to physically get together and many people are comfortable with using social media. If we can ensure that people also physically meet and bond, then social media, like an online group or a practice intranet, can be a useful way for people to 'bump into each other' virtually. Through this, people can help each other, share ideas and opinions, be light-hearted, laugh together and so on, all of which help people to feel that they belong.

One caveat is that because electronic media do not have rich non-verbal language, they can be a way of 'mis-communicating' and 'mis-understanding'. Our challenge is therefore to use different forms of communication for what they do best, but also to encourage people to interact face-to-face.

Case example

Jo, a new records manager, found that a few of her staff were sending each other emails about work-related issues even though they were sitting close to each other. As a result, they weren't speaking to each other and this needed to be corrected. She made a rule that colleagues should speak to each other instead of messaging wherever possible and this turned the office into a noisier but more connected place.

When people are physically separated, especially at different ends of the same floor, on different floors or in different buildings, the problem is compounded because the less they communicate, the harder it becomes to do so. Their communication skills may also start to atrophy through disuse and we may need to make special efforts to support them as we reconnect them with the wider group.

Additionally, people who are physically separated can feel physically and then emotionally marginalised, especially if their work does not involve them interacting with other people. They can become grumpy and unapproachable and this sets up a vicious circle whereby people who initially don't see them, then don't want to see them.

Seeing and talking to each other is not just a nice idea, it is essential and there are studies that show an inverse correlation between the quality of teamwork and the physical distance between people in a traditional workplace. Virtual groups have issues of their own but predictably, they also struggle to become teams because of the factors we have highlighted.

Using these insights, we can do much as leaders to improve the situation on a daily basis, for example:

- Walking about, so that we see others and they see and talk to us
- Having good room layouts, drinks facilities etc. so that people 'bump into' each other

- Preventing people becoming isolated
- Encouraging people to get up and go to talk to each other
- 'Enforcing' break times where people physically get together for a cup of coffee, lunch, etc.
- Encouraging people to use the kitchen and take breaks in communal areas
- Encouraging communal activities, which can be anything from walking together to the corner shop for a sandwich, to planned social activities or more structured 'team-building'
- Encouraging social media for what it is good at doing

The bottom line is that if people don't come across each other in a conducive way, they can't develop the relationships upon which team-working depends.

Feel safe

Teamwork requires us to share with each other, in particular our energy, ideas, attitudes, skills and commitment. However, although sharing sounds cosy and nurturing it can be a risky business as we could be damaged by our co-workers for doing so. For example, by being made fun of, ridiculed or even censured. Trust between people is therefore essential and as leaders our role is to create a safe environment that promotes mutual respect and allows people to lower their guard and to share.

In this and the following sections, we will explore some of the basics that need to be in place and then how people flower and become increasingly productive by moving from feeling *safe*, through feeling at *ease* to feeling *good*.

Safe foundation

'Feeling safe' is like a house, the foundation of which is that people feel that they have a safe job and a safe income. If these are under threat, the walls of our life can feel like they could tumble down.

Why the accent on job and income? Perhaps because we shouldn't presume people's motivation. Some may have a higher sense of purpose but many, especially employees, come to work for a salary that allows them to do other things in their life that may be even more important to them than their work.

Safe from being taken advantage of

Have you ever tried to motivate colleagues and found that they seem 'resistant'? Sometimes the reason can be that some basic needs, for example, to do with working conditions, haven't been met. These needs, sometimes called hygiene factors (2) are not motivating in themselves, but because they are basic, they can be profoundly *demotivating* if they are not attended to. If not met, people may feel that they are being taken advantage of. We sometimes recognise such needs through the fact that they can lead to low morale, disputes, and people leaving.

Case example

Lucy was the third new salaried GP to join the practice. The other two had left after six months and the practice were anxious to get it right. Lucy shared her thoughts about feeling isolated and not being helped to get to know the staff, to find out who does what and to understand the systems. No individual was to blame but she felt unsupported and was reticent to keep taking her problems to the practice manager. As a result, the practice developed a new process for salaried GPs that included an induction period, a buddy chosen by the new doctor, and regular review meetings. Lucy decided to stay and later went on to become a partner.

Another aspect of not being taken advantage of is working in a system that is seen to be fair. As leaders our task is to make sure that the practice provides conditions at work that treat people with equal respect and prevent them feeling vulnerable where this could be avoided, for example:

- By having fair and transparent processes especially for sickness, taking leave, promotion, performance evaluation and grievance resolution.
- By recognising and dealing with poor performance and behaviour.
- By having clear and transparent expectations of what is required of people.
- By being open and honest in our dealings at all times, especially in acknowledging where we have got it wrong or could do better.

Like job and salary, these issues are very hard for those affected to raise for discussion. A fact of life is that some 'bosses' use that barrier to avoid the discussions that as better leaders, they would be initiating.

Safe to be vulnerable

Beyond those matters that affect us all, each of us is vulnerable in our *own* way. The evidence shows that we are happier and therefore give more at work if we are treated with compassion and have our suffering acknowledged, even when there is nothing that can be done to address the cause. We feel more secure if we know that when important matters like our health, family issues and relationship problems occur, we can discuss these if they are affecting our work.

Knowing that the practice looks out for us, that it 'has our back' and that we will be supported rather than be reprimanded or ignored, is a cornerstone of feeling secure. Of course, there are limits to how much responsibility and support the practice could or should offer, but these can be clarified.

What about ourselves? As leaders, we can help by being open and sharing our own vulnerability, as discussed in Chapter 4, because our behaviour is taken by many as a sign of what is okay, even what one is *expected* to do as part of the shared culture.

Safe to speak up to those more powerful

For most people it can be hard to question, challenge or even disagree and yet for our teams to be creative, we all need to be able to do this. How it's done is of course a different matter. Voicing contrary opinions may sometimes feel uncomfortable when it's with our peers, but it can feel positively unsafe with people who are more powerful than us, for fear of the consequences.

As leaders we can remind ourselves that challenge and dissent, when they are well-intentioned, help our development because they can shine a light on the risks of action or inaction, or can lead on to discussions that generate better options. Speaking against an issue does not mean that people are speaking against the team. However, it can still feel as though such people are being awkward or unsupportive.

Even though we may know in our heads to allow dissent, that doesn't mean that we have it in our hearts to do so. However, if we want our colleagues to speak up, it's really important that we respond to dissent well, as people will watch closely for what our tone of voice and body language are communicating and whether these suggest that although we are saying one thing, we are really thinking or feeling another. We must avoid reprisals, the obvious ones being to take action against individuals. Additionally, we should avoid the *hidden* reprisals that only we would be aware of, such as not helping 'awkward' people to develop and further their careers.

Beyond helping people to speak up, if we can be seen to put those with less power at their *ease*, we can do much to build openness and trust. Let's take this further.

Safe to offer our views

As leaders, we recognise that it's the diversity of thinking and perspectives that fuels our team's creativity. Everyone has a viewpoint and ideas, but many people don't recognise that theirs are potentially valuable. The risk is that their views may not be heard or even be considered worth hearing and we can overcome that by building trust. Trust isn't built on a one-off intervention but is a matter of being persistently proactive in involving people in conversation, asking for their thoughts and showing that these are appreciated.

Appreciation does not always mean acting on those views, because doing so when inappropriate could undermine trust in other ways. However, being heard is perhaps what matters most and in many situations, this may be enough.

Safe not to cover up

As a healthcare organisation, we are a community responsible for a safe approach to patient care, which means that each of us has a duty not to look the other way when we see behaviour and incidents that are of concern, but to bring them to the attention of appropriate colleagues or authorities.

Rarely, this duty may include whistleblowing. Understandably, this feels risky, but our role as leaders is to help our colleagues do their duty and not feel that there is a clash of loyalties that might come back to haunt them. The more the earlier steps of 'safety' are addressed, the fewer the barriers and the easier it is for everyone to do the right thing when it really matters.

How much of what you have just read about 'feeling safe' is reflected by your own organisation and what does that say about the culture of your workplace? We need to be proactive to create a safe environment. If we are not, the things our colleagues want and need to share will not go away but will just come out in less helpful ways.

As an indicator of our cultural climate, might it be that the more that our team has to rely on being *courageous* to share their thoughts, the more open and supportive we need to become?

Feel at ease

Moving on, even when people feel safe, they may not feel *comfortable* because although addressing safety can reduce fear, it takes more than that to help people feel relaxed enough to be open.

Being comfortable with co-workers

People do not have to agree with each other. As we've seen, our diversity is the grit in the oyster that allows the pearl of good team-working to form. When disagreeing, seeing things differently from each other or calling each other to account, it is vital to maintain civility, mutual respect and where possible, treat each other with kindness. As leaders we have an important role in modelling and reinforcing this.

Sometimes people are uncomfortable, not because of interpersonal conflict, but because of really unhelpful or demoralising attitudes and behaviour from their colleagues:

Case example

Natalie loves to be contrary. Whatever someone says, she will tend to give the opposite view. What she says isn't so much a problem as how she goes about it, where she can shout and become aggressive. This makes people cower and feel very uncomfortable.

To describe a couple more negative types, have you come across people who tend to coast and be 'slackers' in the team? Sometimes, they can be clever about it and just do enough not to be spotted by management or picked up for underperforming. Or how about the ones who moan and bring people down, just casting gloom, like a bad smell, about the place?

Dealing with such people is not easy, but damaging behaviour shouldn't just be excused as being 'part of their character'. Personality can't be changed, but behaviour can, and challenging this behaviour and helping people to find better alternatives is part of a leader's role.

On a more positive note, we can use and promote those behaviours, especially in meetings, that encourage people to feel comfortable and to contribute. This can counter some of the damaging behaviour that others might bring.

Being comfortable with power and rank

In Chapters 5 and 10, we look at how the power dynamics between people affect the way they relate. Here, we will focus on rank. Both of these affect the degree to which people feel okay with each other.

In life, rank is everywhere. It applies to almost every human feature we can think of such as height, skin colour, gender, disability, education, housing, wealth, title and so on. We bring it up here because it's one of the great 'undiscussables', an elephant in every room.

Rank is our way of clarifying what our position is within the group and it indicates something about what the social group expect of us and what we feel we are entitled to. It's an indicator of our standing in the community and therefore affects our sense of self-worth. Rank can be problematic when it leads to significant unspoken assumptions about what people's relative importance is, what they are valued for, what they are permitted, entitled to and so on.

Rank is not straightforward. For example, in primary care, we receive mixed signals such as being told that even though there are clear differences in authority and power, everyone is equally valuable. This can cause dissonance and may even feel like a deception.

In our daily lives, we occupy several ranks simultaneously and the differences in rank in our various social groups are an added complication.

So, what can we do about it? Discussing it openly may be all that is possible and may be enough because it can stop important assumptions from remaining hidden. Careful facilitation is required, but the process can be cathartic and can be an important part of fostering openness and honesty in the group. Experience shows that if people in a close community, especially a team, are allowed to talk about rank, it really clears the air. There is a notable sense of ease thereafter and relationships become more comfortable, even when people had not noticed the friction that had previously existed between them as a result of this issue (3).

Another important form of rank difference between people is education. In primary care this is significant because people work very closely together and the differences in education and qualification between them can be extreme. Clinicians may not appreciate how this makes others feel, but a relative lack of formal education can be a real barrier to how comfortable people feel about volunteering their thoughts. As so often in these situations of disparity in power, position and influence, it falls to those with more to help those with less, to feel included and valued. It's another manifestation of respecting each other, respect being something that colleagues come to feel, not through what we profess but through how we behave.

Being comfortable and understood through openness

There's also a sense of ease through feeling that whatever the issue, it can be discussed and that those who 'name the elephant' will not be victimised. The issues we've covered here, conflict and rank, are two good examples. One is obvious the other covert, but both are powerful in their effects and have wide-ranging and cathartic benefits when they are skilfully discussed. Through being open, we can chip away at the façade that prevents us being, or being allowed to be, our genuine selves both as individuals and consequently, as a team.

Over the stile

In this chapter we've considered how people who work in the same organisation can learn to open up and relate so that they work well *with* each other rather than just alongside each other.

Safety, trust and mutual respect are a start and attending to them creates the conditions that unlock the energy and motivation that we all have. As we cross the stile, in the next chapter, we will build on this foundation and look at how we help people to connect with what they care about and in so doing, feel sufficiently motivated and valued.

References

1. West, M.A. (2012). *Effective Teamwork: Practical Lessons from Organisational Research* (3rd ed.). John Wiley & Sons and the British Psychological Society. ISBN: 978-0-470-97497-1.
2. Herzberg, F., Mausner, B., & Snyderman, B. (1959). *The Motivation to Work* (2nd ed.). New York: John Wiley. ISBN: 0471373893.
3. Mr Edmund Cross, Facilitator of Professional Team and Organisation Development, personal communication, May 13, 2019.

14

Energise and motivate

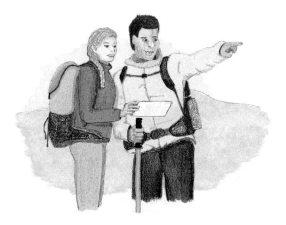

In this chapter, we will explore these questions:

- Where does our motivation come from?
- How can we achieve a balance of motivators?
- What is the place of rewards?
- How might people become aware that they matter?

Feeling motivated

What does motivation suggest to you? A look at the dictionary will show that many of the synonyms for motivate, like drive, propel, spur and so on suggest that motivation is to do with being energised.

People sometimes talk about motivating others and even regard it as their responsibility as leaders and managers to do so. However, because major sources of motivational energy come from within, perhaps we need to think less about what we do *to* people than about what they can do for themselves in harnessing their inner energy. Our task becomes getting to know our individual colleagues well enough to understand which of the motivators for change that are described below could be employed for each of them.

As individuals become energised, the team becomes energised.

Our motivators for change

Let's imagine that we have defined an improvement task. Once we have got an appropriate group together, we will need to harness their energy.

The following diagram shows five major areas of motivation which we will discuss. Between them, these areas cover many basic desires, such as the need for approval, to learn, to experience loyalty, to have friends, and to have social standing. It is unusual for any one motivator to be sufficient in itself. They are synergistic and give us a number of ways of getting people on board with changing things for the better.

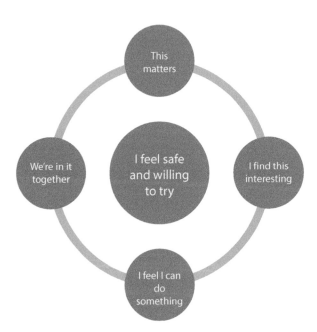

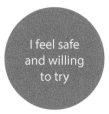

We will address this first because it's like a final common pathway. It doesn't matter if the other motivations have been addressed; if people don't feel 'safe and willing to try' then those motivations will be blocked from having an effect. What's our role in facilitating this? Most importantly, it is to attend to the areas we discussed under 'feeling safe and feeling at ease' in Chapter 13.

Beyond this, there are other factors too. People feel energised if they believe that the effort that they put in will lead to results. In other words, they feel that the task is both feasible and will be used to make a difference and therefore, it is not a waste of time to try.

Of course, people are much more willing to try if they know they will be rewarded for their efforts. Rewards are powerful and could come from external sources like a bonus or from something as simple, immediate and important as recognition and appreciation.

The reward could also come from their internal motivation, such as the human need to develop or to be valued by the people with whom they work.

Few things motivate more than feeling that a task is important and worth-while. It could be that the task matters to people personally because there is a bonus attached, but the deeper feeling that we are doing something that is valuable to the community is even more energising. Leaders can stimulate this by helping people to feel that what they do makes a difference and this is done in part by making use of inspiration.

As discussed in Chapter 3, inspiration is valuable because it energises and makes people less fearful. We can encourage people to notice the feeling of inspiration and to act on it quickly, perhaps by coming to us for support, rather than letting it fade.

As leaders we can help keep inspiration alive. For example by showing how progress with the task, particularly around making life better for people, is helping to deliver something meaningful to the team. Narrative is powerful and we can use stories that describe how team members have done something tough by overcoming barriers, risks, personal fears or anxieties, to make things happen. These small everyday tales of courage really inspire the community.

Case example

Setting up a new call-handling pathway designed for the reception-ists to implement, involved a huge effort. However, the practice collected and shared data on access times, which showed how these were improving. As a result of this feedback, along with the positive comments from patients and much higher ratings for the practice, the team's energy for implementing the change was maintained and morale was kept high. Alongside this, sharing small stories of indi-viduals who had been courageous in dealing with difficult situations, or who had overcome a lack of self-confidence in using their initia-tive, did much to inspire colleagues.

People feel energised when they understand *why* a change is necessary. There has to be a good reason, and to be compelling the reason needs to be important and clear. In addition to whether it matters, people are also energised when they feel intellectually *stimulated*, and one method is to encourage colleagues to develop new insights and to be creatively engaged in problem-solving, as we discuss in Chapter 18.

People are motivated when they don't feel like an insignificant cog in the machine but believe that *they* have something valuable to contribute to a task that matters to the group. We can nurture this in a number of ways. For example, by supporting them and stretching them to develop, by help-ing them to plan goals that are achievable and by giving clear and timely feedback about their effectiveness. They can then use this to improve their performance in-task rather than after it.

We can also help them to develop a sense of agency (personal control) by encouraging them to monitor their performance, pick up on errors and work on them.

Motivation is important, but so is ability, because low ability can't be made up for by any amount of motivation. We can assist people by helping them to acknowledge an 'ability gap' and by providing the resources and training to address this.

In addition, with all of these interventions, we mustn't forget the importance of encouraging people through positive feedback on their efforts.

We're in it
together

In some ways, this can be the best part of being a member of a good team; the feeling of closeness, belonging and a sense of pride in what the team does. As leaders, we can foster that by helping people to get to know each other at work and socially. This helps them to go beyond being a group, to becoming a team in which they care about each other and provide mutual support. We can also nurture high performance and solidarity by giving recognition and reward to the team for what they have achieved *together*. This can be even more powerful than giving recognition for individual contributions, although this is also important.

It's a misconception that good teams are necessarily happy all the time as the best teams often forge their strongest links through adversity. Our role as leaders might be both to raise awareness of this so it doesn't come as an unpleasant surprise and to help facilitate the difficult conversations that allow individuals to be open with each other.

We also have ways of helping the team to grow:

Case example

The data management team had been performing well and Barrie, the practice manager, gave them unexpected feedback. He said he was pleased with them and then gave them a much more difficult task, which was to design a new system of automated referrals for the doctors to use. He said he would not have asked this, but they had demonstrated great ability and he knew that they had it in them to excel. Put across in a different way, being given a further task for completing the original task, could have seemed like a punishment. However, his 'magic feedback' did the opposite of demoralising them.

'Being in it together' for our teams is actually about commitment to each other and relates both to our strengths and our vulnerabilities. We value each other for what we are capable of and this encourages drive and competition. However, our vulnerability also helps us to connect and can bring us together even more strongly. Is that something that you have noticed, perhaps with colleagues you found difficult until vulnerability provided an opportunity for you to connect?

Even if someone is temporarily unable to contribute and be useful to the team's task, they still matter to the team. The highest performing teams may therefore be less like happy families and more like a war time 'band of brothers'.

Getting a balance of motivation: a fingerprint for success

The forms of motivation that we have described are not independent but reinforce each other and it seems helpful not to neglect any of them but to work towards some balance between them. Have a look at the diagram below, which shows a situation in which the balance is problematic. We could use this as a tool that gives a fingerprint for the motivation of the team and helps us identify where we should intervene.

Let's consider this example.

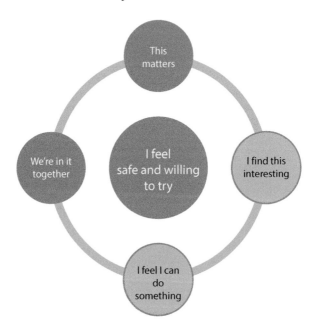

In this team, the motivations of 'I find this interesting' and 'I feel I can do something' are high (i.e. not problematic) and the others are low. People understand the reason for change and also have a sense that they have something to contribute. However, the lack of solidarity or feeling that what is being suggested actually matters, will undermine the team's efforts to move forward. Because people don't feel engaged with change, they don't feel psychologically motivated and keen to try.

This quick overview gives us an early warning that the team will not gel and that the task will fail unless we take steps. Alerted by this, we might explore with the team how and why the task matters to the community and connects to our shared values. This might help the team to feel more unified and more motivated to try.

Working out what motivates

In addition to the *team* fingerprints, each of us has our own *personal* fingerprint of what motivates us, and we can use this to identify our needs and drives. As leaders we can become aware, particularly through socialising and finding out more about people's personal lives and hobbies, of what motivates them. This can be really useful when we come to convene a team for a particular task. For example, it can be helpful to know who amongst our colleagues:

- Likes the work to be challenging
- Likes to be popular
- Always wants to lead the group
- Enjoys controlling people
- Becomes bored when doing routine jobs and so on

Rewarding people and keeping the motivation going

Motivation may be powerful but even intrinsic motivation can't be sustained without recognition and reward. Further than that, *not* doing so is not a neutral act, as a persistent lack of recognition and reward can leave people feeling crushed. People leave if they don't feel valued so the financial as well as the human cost of getting it wrong, is considerable. If such people *don't* leave and we do not remedy the situation, it can be even worse as we end up working with colleagues who are resentful and disengaged.

So how could we do this better? The best rewards are not always financial but are personalised, meaningful and reinforce the culture and values of the practice.

In the Sandybrook practice, the practice manager bought a simple rubber bath toy which she called the golden duck. There was a whiteboard in her office on which anyone in the team could nominate a colleague for going above and beyond, stating what they had done. Every week, all of the nominees were congratulated and a winner was selected. The duck became a much-coveted prize and those who had won three times were given a gift voucher. The fun, inclusiveness and democracy of the golden duck did much to improve morale and camaraderie.

Giving people clear and public recognition for their contribution makes an enormous difference to their self-esteem and powerfully reinforces the positive culture of the practice.

There are many other good ideas for rewards beyond a pay bonus. Here are a few:

- Concert or theatre tickets/gift card
- Early release from work/work from home day
- Team lunch/team movie
- Personalised mug

Case example

Michael had worked hard on producing an induction package and programme for new health care assistants. As a thank you, the practice purchased two guitar lessons for him. He was particularly touched, because he had not talked about his interest in the guitar very openly and people had clearly gone out of their way to find out what he cared about.

Feeling happy

Next, let's think about happiness and how this connects to motivation. There is an interesting representation of this which the Japanese call Ikigai, meaning one's hopes from life. An interpretation of this is shown below. One insight that it offers is the importance of making the connections by trying to find out what people love, identifying what the practice needs and then making sure that people have the skills to apply what they love in a way that benefits the practice. The challenge for us as leaders is whether we just accept this as theory or whether we are prepared to make the sustained effort that can make this route to happiness a reality. What's *our* motivation in doing so? Maybe it is that if we succeed, there is no limit to what people with this degree of fulfilment can achieve.

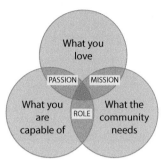

Feel we matter

Encourage both uniqueness and belonging

We touched on this in Chapter 6. Everyone needs to feel that they are not a 'number', in other words that they have something individual and unique to offer the team. Our skill as leaders is in recognising unique attributes that are useful to the team and bringing them in for the benefit of all. Very often, these attributes are not something that helps the *job* of primary care. This isn't surprising, because it would be unusual for an individual to have a skill that no one else possessed. However, what uniqueness can help is team-working. For example, some aspect of how teams define their purpose, values and how they work effectively together. All these factors shape the culture of the practice.

> ### Case example
>
> Ross is quiet and hardworking but has a dry sense of humour which he uses to poke fun at situations and tease people in a kind but never in a damaging way. We encourage this in Ross, because we recognise that his ability to make people laugh is invaluable in defusing tense situations.

As leaders, we can reinforce how uniqueness is valuable to the team by recognising and applauding it. For example, we might thank a particularly conscientious receptionist for coming in early and getting the shift off to a good start, thereby helping everyone to have a better day.

Our colleagues not only need to feel different and special, they also need to feel a sense of acceptance and belonging. Part of the way forward is to create a climate in which people's differences are recognised, talked about, valued and made use of. This process challenges our prejudices and makes us less likely to be dismissive or antagonistic to those who are different from us.

Case example

Zara is a transgender receptionist who was originally male but is transitioning to a female identity. This was the first time the practice had to deal with such an issue and many people felt uncomfortable, not just about the issue but about their ignorance and worry about doing the wrong thing. Zara faced some teasing initially, but after discussion with the senior manager whom she trusted, she helped to set up an in-house learning event which was very well received. Not only did staff feel more comfortable, but they respected the difficult journey Zara was on, and supported her. Although patients were not officially informed, it was noticeable that young people started consulting about gender identity issues and the practice came to be seen as a vanguard in this area.

Over the stile

Connecting people to their motivation, rather than making assumptions or hoping that what we do as leaders will energise them, is a challenge and takes significant effort. If we do it well, the team powers itself to a large degree. However, being energised and having the will to collaborate doesn't mean that a group of relative strangers will work well together.

As we move on to the next chapter, we will consider the assistance leaders can give as teams apply their energy to both challenge *and* co-operate with each other in working towards a common goal.

15

Lead the team to be their best

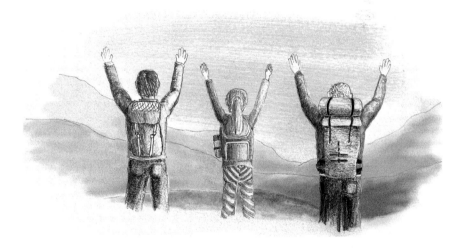

In this chapter, we will explore these questions:

- How can we build and support a new team?
- What phases can we anticipate a team passing through or returning to?
- How can we facilitate the team so that these phases are manageable?
- How can we gauge the team's performance?

Which building blocks do we need to create the team?

We need the right people for the job

Because the task defines the team, once we know what's required in broad terms we can recruit the right people. However, herein lies an issue, because there is an assumption that we know the strengths of people in the community from whom we are selecting. As leaders, we need to be on the lookout for talent and additionally, make plans to assess how individuals perform so that we can develop our pool and have more choice.

It is relevant to know people's personalities and interpersonal skills. These are important to team-working, but they shouldn't be a barrier that limits our choice. For example, if people have the appropriate knowledge and skills but lack the ability to relate well, then working in a team if properly supported, can be a powerful way to develop the skills needed for collaboration.

Teams that function well are small, usually fewer than ten people, and also have an appropriately diverse mix of people with knowledge and skills that are different, but that also overlap. These overlaps are important because they can stimulate connections between people in the team and thereby improve the joint capability of the group. The overlap of our primary colours as discussed in Chapter 5 is an example of this.

Like a coin, diversity has two sides. It is good for creativity, problem-solving and skill-mix, but it might also increase the potential for disagreements and conflict. Being aware of this allows us to anticipate and manage teams in ways that we will now discuss.

Supporting them so that they can give their best

Being part of a team is risky, because team members are trying to meet a challenge and are exposed by being in the public eye. As leaders, we can support them in several ways. First, we should make sure that they feel cared about through listening, learning and taking concerns seriously.

Second, we can fight the team's corner, for example, by making sure that the team has the resources it requires to do the job, such as money, training and technology. At a personal level, we might also provide emotional support, practical help and coaching.

More specifically, we can explore their motivation and try to engage their energies as discussed in Chapter 14. Our behaviour in helping our co-workers sets the tone and encourages team members to help each *other*, rather than just depending on the leader.

What approach might we use?

There are many models that give us insight into the approaches that can be used. The table below is drawn from Hersey and Blanchard [1] and is useful in showing that teams naturally vary in their competence and commitment. This is partly related to the experience they have and how mature they are as a group. The characteristics of new groups are shown at the top of the table, progressively going down to the most experienced groups at the bottom. This model can guide us when we are trying to get the best out of the team, for example by giving us the confidence to *instruct* inexperienced people and conversely, to have a *light touch* with people who are experienced and skilful.

HOW COMPETENT ARE THEY?	HOW COMMITTED ARE THEY?	OUR LEADERSHIP APPROACH
Unskilled, new to this	Willing to learn	Tell
Semi-skilled, inconsistent	Unmotivated	Coach
Skilled and consistent	Reliable and confident	Delegate
Experienced and skilful	Lacking in confidence	Support

How could we help the team to work well together?

Some authors, particularly Tuckman [2] and Wheelan [3] have suggested that groups develop in defined ways, passing through a number of predictable stages. Others have challenged this and suggested that in a complex world, groups of people do not pass sequentially through stages such as forming, storming, norming, and performing.

Instead, the stages can happen in different orders and some stages may be re-visited. For instance, when functioning groups are destabilised such as when there is a change in team membership, they may go back to the storming phase where the balance of power between new and existing members is again contested. If differences can be resolved stability can be re-established, although as we can now appreciate, because situations change this will never be long-term.

One useful insight is that in order to function well, teams *have* to go through periods when they are at odds with one another. This is helpful to know because it stops us from expecting harmony and productivity from the outset. Disagreements between people are not necessarily a sign of being dysfunctional, but may be a sign of strength if the group puts those differences to good use, such as in being creative together. We will see examples of this in Chapter 18.

So instead of talking about stages, which implies a predictable progression, we will think here about the *phases* in which teams find themselves. As leaders this helps us to be more open-minded and notice the phases that we actually see, rather than search for the stages that we expect to see. By doing this, we can tailor our assistance appropriately. Let's consider these phases and as you read on, think about your own teams and which phases you have (and have not) recognised in their development.

As leaders, how can we help our teams in the following phases?

When they come together

Teams are all about the people and the task, so let's first think about the people. It's unlikely in our practice that the team members will be unknown to each other. They may well have worked together in the past and we may know quite a lot about their personalities and how they get on with each other. Indeed, this may have been a significant factor in deciding the membership of the team.

People will need to get to know each other well enough so that they can trust each other, make mistakes together and be mutually supportive so that they reach their goals. Our 'people focus' in this phase will be around facilitating conversations, helping people to open up and share their concerns and expectations, especially around who does what. Socialising is great for developing relationships, and we may play an active part in encouraging that.

We may also establish the ground rules for how people communicate and relate to each other, particularly regarding any conflicts and disagreements and any confidential information that is shared. This is important because it gives people security and shouldn't be assumed. It's rare but not unknown, to have a formal agreement about the team's code of conduct. Chatham house rules are an example of this, whereby the source of information disclosed in a group cannot be shared without permission. Mostly though, we can establish the ground rules and set the tone in clear but more informal ways.

Everyone will be interested, even anxious, about the nature of the task. Therefore, a very significant part of our role at the start is to clarify the purpose of the team and the contributions that are expected, i.e. the task, the goals and the roles and responsibilities of team members. Additionally we may clarify how decisions are made, the lines of accountability and of course the timeline for the project and when we are expecting to see signs of progress. Being clear about the goals may involve us in being more directive and 'telling' people more than 'discussing', but this is needed because teams quickly lose confidence if they don't know exactly what is expected of them. To give a deeper insight, task or project management is discussed in Chapter 23.

Not everyone is enthusiastic about change and negative thoughts are a natural reaction that we should expect. We can help take the sting out of the change process at the start by not making assumptions and by creating a safe space in which people can say:

- What they are concerned about
- What is good about what they are *currently* doing that they wish to preserve
- What they are concerned about losing as a result of the change and so on

In doing so, we model the importance of openness and honesty in the group, give people the opportunity to say the unsayable and thereby lessen problems down the line.

Because the project team will be the very people who sell the change to colleagues in our primary care community, it's particularly important that they are helped to do so. We can assist, for example by providing opportunities to give feedback on progress at meetings, on posters or through the intranet. We can also help individuals to become better communicators.

Rarely, the nature of the project may be such that the team are not clear at the start about the specific tasks. For example, a new team coming together to form a primary care network with representation from each member practice. In such circumstances, leaders can facilitate them to consider their purpose, aims and goals. From these, the tasks will become clearer.

When there is conflict between team members

As we noted, this phase is not avoidable and if we appreciate how disturbance makes us stronger, this can help us to manage our own discomfort as well as that of the team.

Generally speaking, this phase comes when members feel that the ice between them has been broken, allowing them to go beyond being polite and to start discussing deeper and more substantive issues like differences of opinion. They might also engage in power struggles, such as competing with each other for the acceptance of their ideas or for the dominance of their role. Like water, people find their level with each other and our role as leaders is not to interfere with this but to facilitate it so that people can challenge safely, work through their issues in a timely manner and still respect each other at the end.

We use a range of skills to do this. We encourage people to listen to each other and respect differences. Using our awareness of how people are behaving, we may need to close some people down so that they don't dominate or control, and encourage the quieter or more introverted ones to open up. We may need to coach some team members to become more assertive and others to become more effective listeners.

Conflict is a difficult word because it tends to make us think about people's personalities rather than the issues that they are disagreeing about. Therefore, to encourage a more objective view, it can be important to depersonalise the situation, clarify the issues and where the disagreements lie and then ensure that these are heard by all parties.

If the conflict is actually of a more personal nature, for example between a couple of members of the team, we may need to pick up on this in private with the people concerned, rather than try to deal with it in the group.

In the rare situation when teams cannot move past personal disagreement and conflict, we still have the option of reconfiguring the team. Of course it's uncomfortable to do so, but we can make it easier by reminding ourselves that the main priority is not the feelings between people in the team but rather, the completion of the task.

When people are settled with each other, but not yet delivering

This is an interesting period during which people are starting to think beyond their own issues and are increasingly considering the needs of the team and their joint work together. They have sufficient respect for each other to be functional and our role is to build on that and help them to create stronger emotional bonds and feelings of trust between each other.

In terms of our power and control, this is an appropriate time to be gradually handing over responsibility while still being ready to step in and take the reins when and if the team get stuck. We can do this by encouraging them to problem-solve and make decisions. We can help them to feel comfortable in making mistakes, and this is fine provided they know not to hide what they believe we may not want to hear, but instead be open with us without fear of recrimination.

We can make this an experience that isn't just about working, but about sharing the risks, rewards and learning that come from experimenting. More specifically, we encourage the team to be courageous, more open, more aware of each other's strengths and better able to learn from each other.

There is anxiety during this phase, because the group has not yet achieved any significant goals and therefore has not yet had the experience of showing competence through delivery, which is so necessary to developing their confidence.

Knowing that, we can help the team to be motivated and develop a good reputation with their peers by planning quick wins, which are short-term feasible goals that demonstrate to the team and to others that they are on track. We can create milestones and make sure that when these are achieved, people are given recognition and reward in order to build their self-esteem and further fuel their motivation.

When they are working well together

This is a golden period when the team is functioning at a high level. They have strong motivation and when there are disagreements, they have good-enough relationships and skills to allow them to work through these and still get the job done.

For a high-functioning group, our role as leaders involves using a lighter touch. We keep things steady, monitor progress and watch for any signs that the team are going off track. There is little if any need for us to solve problems or make decisions on their behalf. In fact, this could be counter-productive. We can also encourage the team to celebrate their milestone achievements and help them to see *how* they have developed their skills both at the personal level and team level.

There is another angle on 'functioning with ease'. Given how pressured life in primary care can be, it may seem odd to talk about 'coasting'. However, coasting might happen when teams are working smoothly and quickly because they are doing things in the 'same old way', not because this is the best way, but because they have slotted into a routine and haven't considered the need for change.

To give an example, a team of administrators may have learned to deal with incoming mail in a timely way by sorting and sending to various clinicians to read and file. However, there might be a better way to handle the process in which the team learn to scan documents and then where guided to do so, read and file these themselves rather than passing them straight on to clinicians.

Leaders can be on the lookout for such opportunities. However, routines are welcome, comforting and in many instances, necessary. There isn't a natural incentive to move out of them and some may feel that 'coasting' is the reward that they have earned for 'getting it right'. And yet, there may still be a need and a possibility for change. Do those sentiments sound familiar to you from the real world of leadership?

When we're not happy with their performance

Here, we will not discuss how we manage poor performance, as this will depend on the circumstances. As with clinical care, diagnosis is often the key, so instead we will consider how we might identify poor performance in the first place.

Let's first consider the individual team member. The early signs of someone struggling to accept the responsibility of their role in the team could include avoiding the challenge, not using their initiative or missing agreed deadlines.

They may also show poor performance in the way they relate to their colleagues. For example, they may blame others when things go wrong, be a gossip, be a 'downer' on the team, show apathy or avoid engaging with other people.

Our first approach is not to punish people, but to try to find out the causes and address them. For people to perform well, they depend upon having clear tasks, adequate resources, encouragement and the opportunity to work without being micro-managed.

If we now think about the performance of the *whole* team rather than just the individual, the picture is broader than just delivering the task. There are a number of other elements and in the table below [4] we show these, alongside a few criteria that give us a flavour of how we recognise good performance and therefore spot its absence in the team.

If we have an issue with an individual, this table also helps us to think more broadly and establish whether there might be factors beyond the individual that could be affecting the whole group.

TEAM FUNCTION	SIGNS OF GOOD PERFORMANCE
Task and goals	These are well understood, accepted and delivered
Commitment and accountability	Team members take the tasks seriously and regard each other as being accountable
Communication	Good participation, people talk to each other, not just to the leader and there is good discussion outside meetings
Conflict	Team members talk about issues, not personalities; people feel comfortable to air their differences and disagreements
Organisation	Meetings are well-prepared and run; they are productive and decisions are jointly-owned
Decision-making	Decisions are well-informed and there is an agreed mechanism for making them
Vision	The team have a vision and are inspired and energised
Environment	There is a no-blame attitude, risk-taking is encouraged and mistakes are used as opportunities to learn

When we *are* happy with their performance

In this pleasing situation, recognition and reward are appropriate and necessary. We considered these in Chapter 14, but here we take note that a key feature in rewarding a team is to have a fair system. Of course, fairness does not mean equality and it's important to tailor recognition and reward to the person and the contribution. For example, it could be seen as unfair and demotivating if everyone received the same reward, irrespective of whether they were a prime mover, someone who did more than asked or just did enough to get by.

Over the stile

We've looked at how team members come together and develop the relationships and skills to give of their best. For leaders, the process has parallels with parenting, not in a condescending manner but in the way our efforts help the team move from anxiety and reliance on external people such as leaders, to a growing state of self-confidence and independence.

We'll now take the next step and consider how leaders and teams move from independence to resourcefulness. In particular, how they use this to adapt and survive, knowing that situations change and that the only certainty is that further difficulties will lie ahead.

References

1. Hersey, P., Blanchard, K.H., & Johnson, D.E. (2008). *Management of Organizational Behaviour: Leading Human Resources.* Classiques Hachette. ISBN: 9780132617697.
2. Tuckman, B. (1965). Developmental sequence in small groups. *Psychological Bulletin* 63(6), 384–399.
3. Wheelan, S. & Hochberger, J. (1996). Validation studies of the group development questionnaire. *Journal Small Group Research* 27, 143–170.
4. Mullins, C. & Constable, G. (2007). *Leadership and Team Building in the Primary Care.* p. 113. London, UK: Radcliffe. ISBN: 978-1-84619-105-3.

16

Adapt and survive

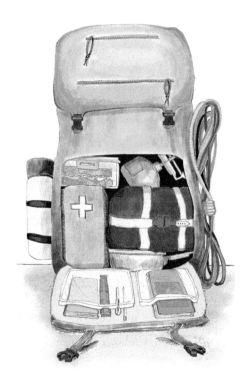

In this chapter, we will explore these questions:

- How are adapting and being resilient related?
- What is the relationship between pressure and stress and how can we protect ourselves?

- What steps can we take to promote our well-being?
- What attitudes help us to see things differently?
- How can the team become more adaptable?
- How can we manage an emergency?
- How can we manage and survive a full-blown crisis?

Help each other over the obstacles

We've come a long way in learning about ourselves, our teams and how to work effectively together. Leaders are needed when situations are unclear and the best way forward is unknown, but not unknowable. One of the most important attributes of good leaders is the ability to facilitate *adaptation* to the situation, which might mean adapting to the problem, the context, the people and usually, all three.

This book uses the metaphor of a hike. Just as when we go walking, leaders expect conditions to change and we can prepare ourselves beforehand and adapt ourselves during the journey as the situation requires.

In this chapter, we will assume that we have the personal skills and abilities to work together that we described earlier. We will focus on how we can remain effective, no matter what the weather.

Walk in a group

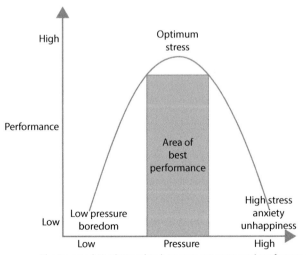

The Inverted-U relationship between pressure and performance

Much of this chapter reflects aspects of 'resilience', especially how we confront stressful experiences and manage them effectively. It's about being hit sideways and responding not just by coping, recovering or bouncing back, but by adapting and growing as a result of that experience.

No significant problem is ever dealt with entirely alone. Resilience is therefore not just the property of ourselves as individuals, but of our group because we each carry different things in our backpacks. Therefore, as we consider the ways in which we adapt to adversity, we will discuss not just how we can personally become more effective but also what we can do to improve the capability and resilience of our team.

Protect ourselves

We know that at some point it's going to rain, or worse, and it would be foolish not to plan for that and have some protection. Life as a leader is rewarding, but it's undeniably stressful. Not only do we have to cope with our own feelings and live up to probably quite high expectations of ourselves, but we also have the weight of other people's expectation to bear. Let's think about stress for a moment, and consider how it relates to pressure.

In the graph shown below, which is based on Yerkes-Dodson's law [1] relating arousal to performance, we can see that pressure is not in itself a bad thing. In fact if we don't have enough of it we become bored, lack stimulation and fail to perform at our best. For example, we know from experience that it can be useful to have a deadline that focuses our attention by applying a healthy, but unremitting, degree of pressure. However, if we have too much of it, that pressure goes beyond what we can cope with and becomes experienced as excessive stress. This is both unpleasant and unhealthy if it is sustained or too intense. Our ideal would be to aim for a life in which there is sufficient pressure, but not too much stress.

By pushing the curve to the right, we find that we are able to tolerate greater levels of pressure and still maintain performance, without feeling this as unhealthy stress. So how do we achieve that? The short answer is by using all the mechanisms discussed in this chapter, which revolve around protecting ourselves, having helpful attitudes and the skills to deal with problems.

Here are a few more specific thoughts on how we can protect ourselves.

Maintaining our health

This sounds obvious, but we know how common it is to neglect this, especially when we are younger and physically more resilient. Prevention is far better than cure.

As health care workers and particularly as leaders, we live lives that feel very busy. This can deceive us into assuming that we are physically active and are taking exercise, but a step counter might show how different this assumption is from reality.

People may burn the candle at both ends and neglect to get enough sleep. This particularly applies to those who like leaders, are driven. Keeping a record over a representative fortnight can show whether we fall into this category. Just one hour short each day would amount to the best part of two nights sleep over the fortnight.

Also, eating well and not skipping meals or having lunch on the run, can help to build the foundation that makes us better able to cope with pressure. In addition to prevention, we need to become adept at managing stress by anticipating it, recognising the early signs and doing things to relieve it.

Although beyond the scope of this book, the importance of psychological well-being cannot be underestimated and this needs our almost daily attention.

Organising

Having too many tasks to do in the time we have available can be a significant and common source of stress for many leaders. The hike analogy might be useful here. If we know we walk at about 3 miles per hour across country and yet we plan a 40-mile trek for the day, it should be no surprise that we will really struggle, possibly dangerously so. Getting better at judging how long we need to do something important can help us with time-pressure by anticipating it and making it manageable. It might also make us reconsider whether the task is feasible in its current form.

Many books have been written about time-management, describing the importance of factors such as:

- Having clear goals
- Delegation
- Avoiding re-work

- Avoiding distractions
- Using 'dead time' well (e.g., when travelling)
- Avoiding procrastination
- Scheduling assertively
- Learning to say 'no'
- Breaking big tasks down into short and simple steps
- Rewarding yourself

However, it's important to see the use of time within a wider continuum, because there's no point becoming *efficient* if that time is not being used to make us more *effective*. Therefore, we should first check that what we are spending our time on is the right or best thing to do in meeting our purpose.

Also, can we learn to be 'good-enough' rather than over-egging it so that we can use our limited resources better? The Pareto principle, which states that we can achieve 80% of the potential outcome with 20% of the possible input, is worth learning about as it is applicable to all manner of endeavours. Leaders are often conscientious and one of the challenges is learning to live with the anxiety of doing less than we would normally feel comfortable with. When we find that lesser effort (or more accurately, better-targeted effort) does not end in disaster, we feel reassured to change and live more sustainably.

Many people find that procrastination is an issue. However, this may not be because of laziness or fear but because of a lack of impetus. It can help to plan, because plans generate impetus. Planning can help us to prioritise the goals we should be devoting our time to, the order in which we should be doing things and the time we should be spending on each. The overall effect is to give us a sense of control and therefore of greater confidence, and to stop us putting things off.

Of course, life is never that linear or controllable and there is a balance between organising ourselves and being flexible and open-minded enough to go off-piste. For example, to ditch the day's plans and deal with the unexpected, to step in and help others when needed, or to have conversations that later lead us in new directions and therefore turn out not to have been 'distractions' at all. As we can see, being organised is not a matter of being rigid and can coexist with being adaptable.

Ultimately, life is short and time should be appreciated rather than rushed through; maybe we should worry less about how we spend our time and instead, savour what we are doing.

Using the 'five ways to well-being'

Protecting ourselves includes looking after our well-being and the following helpful advice is drawn from a significant project by the New Economics Foundation.

Connect with people: Invest time in building relationships with friends, neighbours and work colleagues. These people support us through difficulties, provide a range of perspectives that help us to find ways forward and give us the compassionate but honest feedback that keeps us on track.

Be active: Exercise makes us feel good. For example, leave the transport and try short walks, find a form of exercise that we enjoy and that suits our mobility and fitness, ranging from gardening to dancing.

Take notice: Of things that surround us and enjoy them. Try to live 'in the moment'. This is a particular challenge for leaders, as our minds are frequently ruminating on a recent interaction, or considering how to approach the next challenge. We shouldn't forget the 'now' but learn to savour the day, notice the seasons, take time to reflect and foster our curiosity.

Keep learning: This includes learning from our work experiences, including our behaviour as leaders. It also means discovering old interests, taking up something new like a musical instrument or developing skills that are not only fun but make us feel more confident and resourceful.

Give: This helps us to connect to a wider community. It makes us feel energised and fulfilled to see how our happiness is connected to that of the people around us. Giving can be as simple as smiling, or could come through donating our time, money or other resources, perhaps in volunteering or fundraising for a cause close to our hearts.

Applying this to the team

As leaders, we can actively encourage well-being, and thereby resilience, through our own behaviour and also by:

- Encouraging physical activity in the team, walking rather than using transport, going on communal activities such as park runs and so on.

- Helping to develop a more effective network between people by connecting them through tasks and helping them to get to know each other at work and socially.

- Encouraging a charitable mindset, for instance by sponsoring team members in their fundraising or by linking the practice with a particular cause for a year.

- Making visible the acts of kindness that we see from our colleagues. For example, we might make a point of recognising publicly those people who go the extra mile.

- Helping each team member to identify and develop new skills.

See things differently

When the weather changes, it's very easy for us to lose our perspective and sense of direction. However, we don't have to remain in the dark and just as on a hike where we would carry a torch, so in real life we can learn to use our minds to shine the light that helps us to visualise better. This light comes through a number of helpful attitudes, which we will discuss below.

Optimism

This attitude is particularly strongly correlated with the most resilient people and teams, whose characteristics are that:

- Crisis brings out the best in them
- They are confident in their ability to turn bad situations into better ones
- They feel secure and therefore better able to take control
- They are curious and enjoy trying out new things

With our rational heads, we may prefer the self-image of being 'realistic'. However, fostering our innate optimism is important because it releases positive energy that makes us feel better-able to help ourselves and our teams to overcome difficulties. This is beyond what the more neutral energy of 'realism' is capable of.

Optimism like other powerful moods such as misery is like a smell or scent; it pervades the team and is noticed by others. Optimism is not a matter of blind belief and this is because it leads us to experiment, learn and improve our capability. It becomes self-validating and self-reinforcing because optimism makes us more capable, and that capability then makes us more optimistic about the future. Optimism is therefore evidence-based and is neither faith nor delusion.

This is illustrated through the diagram below, which shows how the group might naturally feel about problems (the oblongs) and how the mindset of optimism (the circles) re-frames those anxieties in a positive way. Although not illustrated here, think about how pessimism does the opposite if it goes beyond correcting over-optimism and becomes systemic.

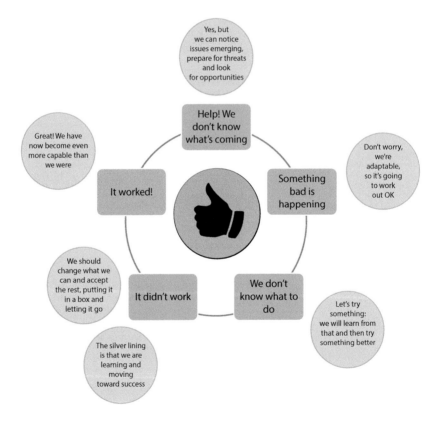

By using the approaches shown in the circles, we can as leaders develop a more optimistic mindset and learn to use it as a powerful tool of adaptability.

Openness and flexibility

Like optimism, these characteristics help us to be adaptable rather than rigidly 'sticking to our guns' with problems or with people. Openness encourages us to be less invested in a particular way forward or be too proud to change. We are more likely to notice what is happening around us and not become blinkered when what we see doesn't fit with what we hope to see. The ability to change course or even do a U-turn, is not a sign of weakness in these situations, but a sign of adaptability, which is a real strength.

We can nurture openness and flexibility particularly by listening, learning and being seen to do so. This connects us more strongly with the team and helps everyone, not just ourselves, to become more confident of dealing with situations that are changing or confusing.

The 3 Ps

The 3Ps model was proposed by psychologist Martin Seligman, who identified three key features about people who show strong resilience. Examples of helpful mindsets in relation to resilience include:

Permanence: We see the effects of bad events as being temporary, not **permanent**. We say 'My team never like my work *on that project*', not, 'My team never like my work'.

Pervasiveness: We don't allow bad effects in one area to **pervade** and affect everything else. We say 'I'm not very good at *this*' rather than 'I'm no good at *anything*'.

Personalisation: We don't always seek a **personal** fault to explain the setback. We say: 'That didn't go well because I didn't have the resources', not, 'That didn't go well because I'm incompetent'. We remind ourselves that it's hard because it's hard, not because we're stupid.

Applying this to the team

We can help our team to become more adaptable by encouraging more helpful attitudes, for example:

- We can behave with confidence and emphasise that even when we don't have answers, as a team we can always find a way through.
- We can't change the event, but we can change our attitude. We can choose not to react negatively or to panic, but to remain calm, keep

things in proportion and find a way forward. We don't need to see ourselves as victims and waste energy on this.

- When we hear negative thoughts in our heads, we can immediately replace them with positive ones like 'I can do this', 'I'm good at my job' or 'I've got over tough things like this before'.
- We can encourage openness, honesty and sharing.
- We can encourage people to talk about the meaning of their work and keep connecting them back to the vision, the 'why', in order to motivate and energise them.
- We can describe explicitly how the team have successfully adapted to challenge. Reminding the team, helps to build confidence and capability for current and future problems.
- Even with positive attitudes and good working practices, not everything is within our influence or control. Look at the diagram below [2]. Within the wide circle of concern, we can focus on those things that we can change which lie within our 'circle of influence', rather than things that are a concern to the practice, but which we can't change and may have to live with.
- For example, we might use this insight in meetings to keep the discussion relevant and constructive, or to discourage colleagues from wasting too much time moaning about 'the state of the world'. As we become more capable, our circle of influence grows wider leading to less frustration, provided of course our circle of concern is not growing at an even faster rate.

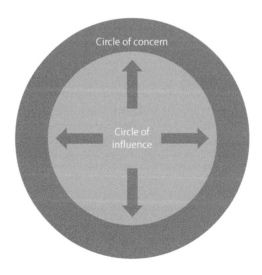

Be adaptable

Be aware and prepare

When we hike, we may take a hat, gloves and scarf. In responding to change-able weather, it isn't just a matter of having the right kit, by which in our leadership context we mean our most helpful attitudes and useful skills. There are also actions we can take in advance to prepare ourselves. Just as with the weather, it pays to take notice of the forecast, what is happening on the horizon and what 'weather' might be coming our way that we could prepare ourselves for.

Some things are predictable, and with good organisational skills we can make our lives easier. The first day back at work after a bank holiday could be a nightmare, but it could be manageable if we planned ahead to have the capacity to take up the strain. Likewise, putting in a new computer system could be made much less stressful if we brought in extra help for a period to give us space, if people were given one-on-one training and if help was at hand from an IT expert in the early period of change-over.

Another form of preparation is upskilling the team to be better placed to take on new opportunities, such as developing minor surgery skills that could then be used by a cluster of practices.

Problem-solving and decisiveness

Like any skill, problem-solving gets better with practice. As leaders, getting people routinely involved in task-based teamwork to improve their problem-solving skills, makes the practice much more able to cope when the less frequent but more serious challenges emerge.

When this happens, it pays to be decisive and make a decision about whether action is needed, sooner rather than later. Simply waiting for the problem to go away only prolongs the crisis. Instead, being decisive gives us a sense of purpose and control. If action is taken, this doesn't have to be the 'best possible'. Spending time trying to develop the perfect plan wastes valuable effort and is probably inappropriate as plans must adapt to evolving situations. Plans and situations shape each other and at the start, what a plan must do is give us a point from which we can act, learn, and improve.

Being decisive and proactive also lets us take advantage of the funds and support that are offered to early adopters to prime new initiatives. Being an early adopter can be a game-changer for the practice by introducing new processes, technology or skills. This helps the process of change to be more manageable and less disruptive overall.

Applying this to the team

- People can lose confidence and become more fearful in bad weather and it takes leadership to encourage a different mindset. We can help colleagues not to feel dispirited by challenges and to view difficult situations as opportunities to find a better path, instead of seeing them as roadblocks. Leaders who convey enthusiasm are, generally speaking, not regarded as being naïve or out of touch, but are valued for being positive

- If we are adaptable, we encourage adaptability in others. If we are inflexible, the team may mirror us in the same way.

- We can share feelings, get support and help the team to come up with positive solutions together.

- The team needs to feel understood and cared about and we can acknowledge the hardships, be compassionate and provide comfort. Being cared about doesn't make the team 'soft', it makes them feel stronger.

- Additionally, we can find things to celebrate and find ways of having fun or laughing at our mistakes *with* the people, not *at* the people involved.

- Adaptation to difficulties doesn't have to be grim. As leaders, we should *have* fun and *be* fun.

- We can give recognition and reward not just for successful adaptation, but for trying and learning. We can take the trauma out of mistakes, failures and complaints by re-framing these. Mistakes are, after all, how we learn.

- We should not just use ways forward that the team are already familiar with. We can encourage innovation as this makes us even more adaptable by doing things differently, rather than just better.

- Adaptation requires courage. By learning to adapt, we become progressively more courageous and learn not to fear the world and think of ourselves as victims, but to experience the joy of having some control.

Respond to an emergency

On our leadership hike, despite our best efforts, emergencies can happen and we can get stuck, injured or lost, at which point our emergency food and drink, first-aid provisions and a mobile phone turn out to be lifesavers. Let's translate this to practice life.

In primary care, in extreme circumstances such as a fire at the surgery or a serious immunisation error that has left many children unprotected from infection, we have to be able to lead from the front. There are some important elements to managing such a situation well.

Keep calm

It is likely that everyone will be anxious and finding things difficult. We will need to use those people closest to us to help us keep balanced and to maintain perspective. In so doing, everyone's stress levels will be reduced.

Take responsibility and show that you care

In some ways, leading an organisation is similar to taking responsibility in a clinician-patient relationship and our ethics can guide us to an appropriate approach. People in the practice, but more particularly the public, will be looking out for signs that we are attempting to avoid responsibility, blame others or trying to cover up.

Therefore, the first step is to take ownership of the problem, admit the emergency, empathise with the pain, inconvenience and frustration being felt and give an undertaking to get to the bottom of the problem and fix it. Even if we don't yet know who or what is to blame, we can publicly express compassion for the suffering that is being caused.

Our legal and insurance advisers will make suggestions aimed at protecting interests, but we should listen more closely to the voices of humanity and integrity, which encourage openness and honesty. In such circumstances, it takes a courageous leader to do the right thing.

Be present, communicate honestly, and communicate often

There should be no knee-jerk reaction and we should pause to make a quick initial assessment and to consult. Being visible is a very important part of keeping the ship steady and this should not be delegated to someone junior or inexperienced. We need to be out there, and seen to be out there, talking to people, finding out the implications of the crisis and supporting those who are working towards its resolution.

Burying our head in the sand is understandable, but there is a steep price to pay for being thought to be indifferent or lacking in courage. It can help to recognise that, as in clinical practice, it is sometimes enough just to let people talk and express their emotions and suffering. A solution in the early stages, may not be expected or possible, but we can *always* show concern and listen closely. We are human and it's important not to put up a façade that hides our vulnerability. If we do, the falsehood is quickly seen and rapidly escalates public anger.

Communicating frequently and keeping people up-to-date applies as much to our team as to our patients. Nowadays, this will happen through a number of channels including especially, social media. Using the phrase 'No comment' is never an adequate response and we also have to remember that over-reacting to an emergency is as bad as under-reacting. Keeping open and balanced is authentic, steadying and sustainable.

Fix the underlying problem

Wherever the problem is coming from, if it's possible to deal with the source, then that should be a priority. In managing the problem, we will certainly have to be flexible and may have to allow normal business to be conducted in abnormal ways, at least temporarily. Interestingly, when we look back, we can often learn important lessons about our adaptability from being forced to do things differently.

Our public relations are critical. If we have shown sincerity, openness and commitment to fixing the problem, the people affected are more likely to be tolerant and forgiving. We shouldn't rely on this or be disappointed if it doesn't happen, as particularly when we have legal liabilities, we must expect the consequences and prepare for them.

Win back trust

Apologies and good communication will hold the situation and prevent it spiralling, but they will not undo the damage. Winning back trust is a slow process, but through showing the commitment to learn and by demonstrating change, relationships can be rebuilt. What we learn from this will help us to be better prepared in the future, perhaps by developing protocols to guide us in potential emergency scenarios.

Applying this to the team

- We need an early warning system. Crises can be detected when they are brewing if our colleagues know to report worrying signs when they are first aware of them. This can't happen without encouragement and by creating a safe space to report, without fear of reprisal for raising the alarm, even if it turns out to be a false one.

- Sometimes, there is a single significant warning such as a near-miss. At other times, there may be recurrent lower-grade events suggesting that a structural problem may exist and that a potential crisis is in the making. For example, repeated fire inspections that point out problems that are then not acted upon in full.

- Colleagues should be encouraged to act with candour and not assume that the problem is already known about or that someone else will pick up on the problem and report it. Our leadership should create a culture in which no one looks the other way. Many times, their interpretation may be wrong, but people should be thanked for raising their concerns rather than burying their heads.

- There are valuable lessons to be learned. What could be a more 'significant event' than an emergency or crisis? When the crisis is over, our colleagues are central to making sense of what happened and learning the lessons that will help us in the future. Rather than just breathe a sigh of relief and get back to normal, a significant event discussion is invaluable and imperative.

- It is also important to acknowledge and celebrate the people and qualities that have helped us to find a way through.

Respond to a full-scale crisis

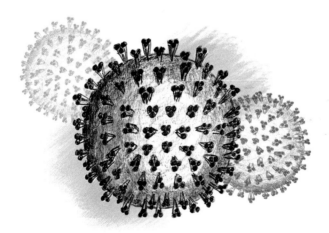

A wider bandwidth of challenge, response and opportunity

Hands up. As authors, we didn't anticipate that primary care leaders would have a personal role in responding to a global crisis. Coronavirus, the world war of our age, changed that view as it has changed so much. However, what we note is that the pandemic not only reinforces the principles of collaborative leadership that we outline in this book but also presents a challenge, and therefore requires a response, that is of greater bandwidth. This response is not just from leaders but from all of society. Hence, how leaders respond to a full-scale crisis is part of a continuum with how they respond to an emergency and this section therefore leads on from the last.

A full-scale crisis, like a hurricane on our leadership hike, is characterised by its scale and speed of progress, which can overwhelm us by making us feel disorientated through our inability to depend on what normally anchors us in life. More than that, our feelings go beyond anxiety and many people experience real fear for their lives and their basic needs.

If there was ever any doubt, the response of societies across the globe shows how important health care is to the citizens of every nation. This brings resources, public support and gratitude, but it also brings expectations of health care workers, who are applauded but are also expected to be heroes in putting their own lives and well-being at risk.

A crisis of this magnitude is an archetypal complex problem. There is no script for how it will evolve and therefore no predetermined plan that we can rely upon. Problems and situations will change quickly, and the way forward will therefore require us to adapt. The risks, for example to people's lives, the economy, social integration and order, are high. However, the opportunities are also great. Whilst working on the daily issues to ensure survival, we can remind ourselves that no such crisis resolves without transformational changes and that because we can expect such changes, we can also influence them.

As always with complexity and uncertainty, how we lead 'people' is as important as how we manage the tasks. Putting in the time and showing the care that builds strong relationships, will pay enormous dividends in a crisis situation.

Be clear, calm and confident

When fear and disorientation abound, misinformation and misinterpretation can make these spiral further. Integrity and competence are the key to maintaining confidence and it is no different in a global crisis. Therefore, openness and honesty matter as never before. We should be clear about what we know, *don't* know and the steps we are taking to find out more.

People need to be appraised of the seriousness of the situation but in a way that doesn't destroy morale. Jacinda Ardern, the Prime Minister of New Zealand, said of Covid-19:

> Every move you then make is a risk to someone else. That is how we must all collectively think. That's why the joy of physically visiting other family, children, grandchildren, friends, neighbours is

on hold. Because we're all now putting each other first. And that is what we as a nation do so well.

This helped to change the public mood and prepare people for the wide-scale sacrifice of liberty. We should neither exaggerate nor minimise the risk or our level of optimism, because to do so will damage credibility and confidence.

Being honest and behaving calmly are important and also powerful when combined with 'measured optimism'. Between them they help us to convey a sense of confidence allied to realism.

When confusion is all around, people need to be brought together, and a clear vision and meaningful goal are invaluable in rallying people and keeping them on track. In Covid-19, the NHS provided something tangible that people could rally around and goals such as 'stay at home to save lives' were powerful because they were simple, practical and meaningful.

As leaders we generate confidence, not by aligning ourselves to a particular solution (e.g. developing a vaccine), but by projecting our complete faith in the people around us who we believe have the passion and ingenuity to overcome anything when acting together. Furthermore, we can reinforce our team's single-mindedness and determinedness by talking about the values that really matter, such as courage, loyalty, and morality.

Safety first

In the coronavirus pandemic, as in any war, a country's first duty is to the safety of its citizens. As leaders, this extends even more so to those members of our team who are fighting on the front line and literally putting their lives at risk. Such people are heroes but should not be *required* to be heroes because the system has let them down through, for example, lack of protective equipment. If we fail to make our team's safety the absolute priority that it is, we will quickly lose trust and undermine the efforts we make to lead our community to a better future.

Show compassion, encourage kindness and gratitude

How does this help? First, in a crisis nearly everyone suffers and people can cope better if they know they are not alone. In particular, they cope better if they feel that their suffering is acknowledged, especially by leaders who take the trouble to talk regularly with the team. Such leaders find out how people are feeling, what is being said and what is *not* being said. They acknowledge how scary things are and they show their appreciation and concern.

Second, these behaviours promote solidarity, a greater understanding of how dependent we are on each other and therefore greater motivation to work together and look after each other, particularly those most vulnerable.

Such attributes, especially compassion and kindness, should be applied just as much to ourselves as to others. Looking after our physical and psychological health as discussed earlier, including acknowledging our own feelings, sharing the workload and using our support networks, helps us to avoid flagging to a the degree that might damage morale. We can help ourselves further by keeping psychologically more buoyant through avoiding too much negative talk and negative people and by thinking positively ('I can do this'). We will try to be prepared but we should also be kind to ourselves when stress and fatigue affect our performance, as they are bound to.

Together, this approach to self-understanding and self-compassion helps us to support ourselves and others whom the crisis has traumatised and exhausted, in a more humane and effective way.

Be decisive, despite the great uncertainty

Unlike in other situations, even emergency situations, it is not possible in a crisis to wait for the best information to emerge. Because of the uncertainty and fear, there is a need to be decisive and thereby show that we are on top of things. If this is not done, confidence plummets despite a leader's integrity or compassion because their competence is called into question. If you want to know how important decisiveness is, just recall how *indecisiveness* feels to those who are being led. To clarify, by decisiveness we don't mean the ability to take immediate action, as just as in clinical practice that may not be appropriate. We mean the ability to make *decisions* quickly and effectively. The decision might be to pause and see what is unfolding and emerging. However, whatever the decision is, it should be relayed quickly and with confidence.

If we cannot wait for the best information, we can at least seek out the best available, and this means looking for credible sources information and opinion on which we can base our decisions. Sometimes, time will not allow for sufficient analysis and reflection, but where possible, we should:

- Pause, using our best information to look at problems from a variety of perspectives.
- Anticipate and take into account what might happen next so that we don't over- or under-react.
- Convey our decision or decision-making process, with minimum delay.

How we convey our decisions and our thinking matters, and doing this well, with sufficient (but not excessive) confidence and resolve, doesn't just augment the faith that people have in us. More importantly, it gives stability to the efforts of many others who put those decisions into action.

Communicate well

Communication is the mechanism by which we share the information that helps us to manage problems and through which we maintain human relationships. Both of these are under the most severe pressure during a global crisis. Good communication can alleviate uncertainty, help people to cope and plan and can show that leaders have some control. Some of the key factors are to:

- *Communicate frequently* which especially early on, might be on a daily basis. It can help to think about each day's communication message in terms of a newspaper headline and ask ourselves 'What is it that people most need to know about *today*?'

- *Make it pertinent and useful:* People will get information (and misinformation) from a multitude of sources but in our own organisations, we can improve the quality of information and guard against people feeling swamped. We can do this by filtering the credible sources, prioritising what people most need to know and translating this into a usable form. For example, national guidelines can be converted to a local 'how to' and local intelligence such as which services are available can be shared and regularly updated.

- *Be visible and available:* This is partly achieved through communication, provided we are also seen, physically and in the media, rather than just read. Additionally, we need to be around, which means that people need to know that we are available and how we can be contacted.

- *Show integrity:* Particularly through openness and honesty such as saying what we know and don't know. In addition, by showing fairness and making sure that no-one is above the rules and guidance that we insist upon for everyone else. This helps to maintain trust and reduce the suspicion which people always have in situations of uncertainty.

- *Be proactive:* In a crisis, doing something is better than doing nothing. This is appropriate when we don't have time to wait for situations to evolve or for higher authorities (which are never as agile) to offer guidance. Because we know our organisations well, we are best-placed to decide on immediate action. In a crisis, this gives us the justification for being proactive and then communicating our actions confidently. By communicating what we do and how this is changing in the light of experience, we show how we as a community are learning, adapting and therefore overcoming.

- *Put things into perspective:* Decisions with serious consequences are being made and we should not make assumptions that people will understand why. Part of our role is to explain the bigger picture and the consequences of doing or not doing. We can also help to maintain a sense of balance, so that we don't take things for granted but appreciate what we have as a community and thereby have compassion for others. This reinforces our values and helps us to maintain our collective morale and commitment.

- *Show concern, compassion and care:* We can ask ourselves: How are people suffering, what do they need, what are they concerned about and how could I respond? We also try to communicate how as a team, we are looking after each other. For example, how we are trying to keep people safe in fulfilling their duties and how we are taking care of those who are suffering, especially those who are experiencing loss or who are grieving. Another aspect of caring is communicating both our appreciation of the many local heroes who go the extra mile and sharing our plans to thank people and reward them, for example, through time off or through bonuses.

- *Improve capability:* Communication isn't just about telling things, it is also about sharing information that helps us to adapt better. For example, we can improve capability by stimulating thinking through sharing people's questions, ideas and solutions. We can also maintain energy and resilience by sharing stories of how we are succeeding, overcoming obstacles and showing courage.

- *Reinforce our vision and core purpose:* Frequently reminding everyone of our 'why?' especially by pointing out how the work that people are doing in the crisis is in line with our values and what we most care about. This helps to maintain our stability and reinforces our optimism and resolve.

Create order where you can

We can't relieve uncertainty through certainty, but we can make it manageable and create some semblance of normality by focusing on those meaningful things over which we have some control. For example, we might do this by organising and delivering such things as help lines, priority services for the most vulnerable, palliative care at home and so on. Creating pockets of order in the system also brings order to people's activity and therefore their lives.

The need for individuals to have meaning and purpose is never greater than during a crisis, as this helps to reduce fear and to focus our minds. As an inspiring example from history, when 'The Endurance' got stuck in the Antarctic ice, Ernest Shackleton insisted that each of the crew continued with their normal duties. He motivated them by reminding them frequently of how and why their work mattered to the wider cause and to each other.

Using leadership in this way helps us as a community to make life manageable for the long haul by occupying, motivating and sustaining us.

Encourage adaptability

As we noted earlier, there is no plan for getting through a crisis and the way forward has to be through collective adaptation. For this reason, other than for setting direction and for specific projects such as quickly building an emergency hospital, top-down or 'command and control' leadership is unhelpful as it relies on compliance rather than experimentation. Many leaders, particularly from other disciplines, feel reticent about relinquishing control as they worry that this will lead to instability. However, complex problems such as a global crisis need the flexible response that instability encourages. Such problems can be engaged with successfully if people have the confidence and resources to use their ingenuity. We explore the mechanics of this in much more detail in the next two sections of the book.

As leaders, we have to create the climate for adaptability, partly by giving permission to innovate but also by creating the expectation that people will experiment. This has to be underpinned by promises of safety, for example, that ideas and concerns can be discussed without censure and that mistakes will be inevitable but must be learned from.

Adaptability needs a clear steer from leaders, which includes setting priorities, asking questions, and clarifying decision-making and accountability. As well as empowering people generally, adaptability also means giving responsibility to the *right* people. Being observant and having an open mind come to the fore in this situation. Some of the people we may choose to empower may not be the 'usual suspects' but those who have shown attributes such as initiative, courage, passion and energy, which make them right for the moment. Such people may continue to be of value beyond the crisis period as we discuss below.

Beyond individuals, crisis adaptation requires teams to work across boundaries and this needs leaders to establish multidisciplinary networks of such teams that can collaborate, coordinate, learn and adapt. In a crisis, it is from networking that most of our rapid learning and innovation arise and its importance cannot therefore be overestimated. As with the teams, leaders will collaborate with each other and where this is done effectively, there may be no need for one individual to take overarching control.

Adaptation in a crisis has to be fast, unlike in usual circumstances. The imperative is to act quickly, taking one day at a time and doing what must be done, rather than what could be done. In a similar vein, meetings that once were planned and lengthy need to become much more frequent, opportunistic and short.

Although all this sounds like a tall order, one lesson from Covid-19 has been the remarkable adaptability of individuals and teams, delivering in a matter of days what previously would have taken years to negotiate and implement.

Our practices and organisations are not so much structures as the people who comprise them, and our adaptation is guided by our values. Therefore, to help us do the right thing in the moment, we could try imagining: what could we look back on as a community that would make us proud of what we did at this time? Or feel bad that we didn't?

Look to the future

Unlike managing an emergency, where our mindset might be that life can return to as it was, albeit with better preparedness for a future emergency, in a full-scale crisis the expectations will be different. Even if the mindset of leaders is conservative, society will not allow 'business as usual' to resume.

Whilst dealing with a crisis, we can also prepare for the future in a number of ways. First, many things will be on hold or delayed such as elective surgery, routine medical reviews, non-urgent investigations, disease-prevention programmes and so on. There will be consequences because of the lack of access to everyday primary care. For example, delayed presentations are likely to have worsened and there will be more psychological and physical morbidity as a result. Also, despite arrangements for contraception during the crisis period, we might anticipate a rise in the birth rate. These examples illustrate that there will be severe workload implications beyond the crisis. However, every crisis will be punctuated by periods of relative respite. This is a vital time for planning, damage limitation, etc., and it can help us to think ahead about how we might use these lulls.

The acute phase of the crisis may be short, but we can't reckon to live off adrenaline for long. We will need to plan to share leadership with key people and consider who will take over leadership responsibilities in the event of exhaustion, illness or worse. We will plan to look after the work-force (which includes ourselves), manage workload and help everyone to remain healthy, particularly psychologically where the damage is often hidden. This will include rota planning so that people have opportunities to recuperate and prevent burnout.

However, despite all these active endeavours, the team will still be strained and weary. Patients will be the same and may also be less tolerant of waiting having already made their personal sacrifices. Their expecta-tions for access and help will have to be managed in line with what the workforce is capable of and, as after a world war, we can expect the period of post-traumatic stress to be prolonged and to need active support.

Second, as well as dealing with the aftermath, we can plan to shape the future. Others within the organisation will help to deal with keeping the ship afloat, but few others will look to the future and the opportu-nities that the crisis creates. We as leaders can do this, and can request assistance from others who are not completely immersed in day-to-day operations.

The time for shaping the future is not after the crisis, when those with power and resources have moved beyond the event, but from the earliest days when we are at our most 'indispensable' and our influence is at its greatest. We will be expected to experiment with new ways of working. This is an opportunity to trial and embed innovation and raise the expec-tation that some proven changes will continue. For example, that 'crisis measures' such as wide-scale online consultations and meetings, or more working from home, should become part of the 'new normal'.

Influencing people is a collective exercise. We are always more powerful together, so creating a network of influence, especially including the vot-ing public, is important in order to lobby those with power.

We can't assume that our value in the crisis is understood, especially when newspaper headlines are more attracted by the obvious importance of such things as ITU beds, ventilators and vaccines. Therefore, part of the primary care leader's role is making evident and publicising the value of their community's work. Whatever the future shape of primary care, it will be critically dependent upon resources. By making our value to the 'war-effort' clear during the period of crisis, there is more chance that primary care will get a fairer share of resources, meaning a bigger slice of the NHS pie.

Lastly, despite the pressures on the team, leaders can use the crisis as an opportunity to improve its capability. As we've noted, more than anything else, the crisis is managed best by those who are adaptable. The crisis needs people to act creatively, use their initiative, make mistakes and learn from them. Knowing this, we can grasp this opportunity to use the crisis to create a safe space for people to express ideas, experiment and to learn from each other. Experimentation doesn't just apply to processes, it also applies to people. By this, we mean that we can experiment with people's capabilities by generating opportunities for them to contribute, by recognising talent and by developing the future leaders within the team.

We can't write a plan to deal with a future crisis, but by improving our capability we will be in a much better place to cope with whatever the future may throw at us, not just in crisis situations, but in the everyday improvement of our services and workplace.

As we noted at the start of this section, a full-scale crisis will demand a wider bandwidth of response. What we have discussed here is therefore not specific to a crisis situation, but is an extension of the attitudes and approaches that good leaders use with their teams on a routine basis. Therefore, what we learn from our leadership in a crisis has the power to help us to become better leaders in all other situations in which we may find ourselves.

Over the stile

As section three of this book draws to a close, we have gained a much better understanding of the team and our role in shaping and caring for a community in which we lead and collaborate.

We now understand a good deal about how to get the best from people, and how to help them and ourselves respond to even the most challenging of situations. Next, as we move forward we will look more specifically at how people engage with the process of visualising and creating change.

As we cross this stile, the next part of the journey is about how people decide on the changes they wish to make, and how they can voice their different perspectives but still bring these into an alignment of purpose that they are jointly able to commit to.

References

1. Yerkes, R.M. & Dodson, J.D. (1908). The relation of strength of stimulus to rapidity of habit-formation. *Journal of Comparative Neurology and Psychology* 18(5), 459–482.
2. Covey, S.R. (2004). *The 7 Habits of Highly Effective People: Powerful Lessons in Personal Change*. London, UK: Simon & Schuster.

4

Our route and destination: Creating a path

Section introduction

We have considered in detail how people can work together effectively on a task. However, to achieve more than can be accomplished through tasks, more perhaps than communities think they are capable of, we must further unlock people's potential. In particular the potential to work on what they believe is meaningful, to use their differences to spark their creativity and to reach consensus despite their different viewpoints and their disagreements.

By combining the abilities that we discussed previously with the unleashed potential that we discuss here, our teams become capable of taking on the baton of leading future changes. In this way, leadership becomes a possibility for the many and not just the entitlement of the few.

Great leaders don't create followers, they create more leaders.

Tom Peters

17

Clarify vision and direction

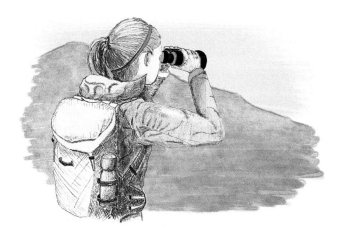

He who has a 'Why' to live for can bear almost any 'How'.

Nietzsche

A key role that we have as leaders is in helping our community establish what is important and what direction we need to move in. Put another way, we help the community to clarify the source of its energy and then help to channel it so that the work the community does, flows from what it cares about most.

There is a sequence here. Clarifying the energy source means helping the community identify what it is moved by, which we might call its *core purpose* and its *core values*. Another term for this is the community's *'vision'*. As we discussed in Chapter 3, one of the most potent sources of this energy is what the group is inspired by and it is therefore useful to help them become more explicitly aware of this.

When the vision is in place, we can channel its energy through work that is guided by *aims and strategies*, knowing that because these are connected to the vision, we are flowing in the right direction.

Vision, aims and strategy, is the sequence that we will therefore discuss in this chapter.

What is vision?

Let's start by saying what it's not. By 'vision', we are not referring to the statements put out by organisations in glossy brochures, which can read like management-speak or platitudes. The very thought of having a 'practice vision' makes some people roll their eyes and suspect it's all claptrap. However, if we appreciate vision for what it can do, the notion is far from trivial.

The vision does not have to be developed often, but when it might be developed is considered below. The problem is that if we don't have a vision, the connection between the aims that carry our energy and their source, may be impaired or even absent.

As a result, the work that we do can become disconnected from what matters most to us and we might find ourselves suffering in a number of ways, including becoming demoralised and exhausted without always understanding why. To give an example, say we have two competing aims, which are to meet patient demand and to provide relationship-based care. We may have to do both but if we just make assumptions and don't discuss our core purpose, we may inadvertently do too much of one and too little of the other and suffer the consequences.

Let's explore a number of facets about vision and how it can be used.

In practical terms, a vision is a short phrase, developed by the team and not owned by an individual, that reminds us *why* what we are doing matters and where we are going with it. It therefore gives us a sense of direction in addition to a sense of purpose.

Leaders are sometimes expected to be visionary. However, more important than the ability to personally describe a vision, is the ability to initiate discussion and clarify what people feel is their purpose, their 'why'. This creates the ownership and motivation that encourages people to collaborate.

Vision connects us to something *bigger* than our current selves, which is why it is powerful, inspiring and makes us *want* to be part of the joint effort.

'Bigger' means higher, broader, deeper and so on, so the language of the vision must open us up to possibilities we may not have imagined and not close us down through being too specific. Some may find this frustrating, but the vision is about enlarging our options for a better future, not about stating how we will bring about change. The narrower 'how' will come later through the aims and strategy, and alerting people to this sequence may prevent them becoming frustrated at this early stage.

As Nietzsche and Sinek [1] have intimated, our vision is our 'why'. Our vision is a reference point that keeps us on track and makes us accountable but very usefully, it is also a tool that we can use to re-energise the team.

As leaders, we do this by talking about the team's work and how our collective achievements connect to our vision. This isn't a one-off exercise, as the process of change is long, so these reminders need to be repeated. Good leaders do it often enough to maintain motivation and momentum but sparingly enough so that they don't alienate people or lessen the impact through overuse. An example is shown in the following table on page 226.

We don't own the vision but we may be the standard bearers who keep the vision in sight, especially in 'battle' when we face obstacles and times are tough. Also, because situations change, our collective vision will naturally evolve so that in addition to connecting people frequently enough to the vision, we also need to periodically re-visit it and ask: 'Are we still doing the right thing?' Finally, a further way of thinking about the vision is as an 'attractor' which pulls people rather than pushes them.

Imagine that we were in Trafalgar Square and wanted to move a large number of pigeons from the margins of the square towards Nelson's column. It would be very hard to push them or goad them into moving in an appropriate direction. However, if we threw birdseed near the column the pigeons would be attracted, almost compelled, to move. Vision is like that bird seed.

When do we need to articulate a vision?

Many practices do not appreciate the importance of the vision and under-standably therefore, do not put time aside to develop one. Doing so becomes important when we:

- **Don't have one already,** in which case the discussion helps to clarify what is important to the team and also brings focus to our leader-ship. Sometimes it can be a revelation to find out how misguided we have been by our assumptions, and it makes us look at our aims in a new light and reconsider whether they are channelling our core purpose appropriately.
- **Need to respond to adversity or to opportunity.** For example, when we are starting a major initiative, wanting to move in a different direc-tion or in any situation where the ethos of the practice might signifi-cantly change. For example, if we are becoming a training practice, are wanting to provide hospital-like facilities in the community or want many more of the team to work from home.
- **Are starting a new organization.** We can think of a primary care network as an example of this. Developing a vision is critical to avoiding assumptions and to helping the network define its iden-tity, its own purpose, values and work focus. This vision, because it reflects a different type of organisation, may well be different from the vision of each of the member practices, but we wouldn't know that unless we talked about it.

In summary, we need a vision when our circumstances change signifi-cantly, because the vision will help us to create a better channel for our energy and will keep our flow strong within it.

How could we develop a vision?

Although leaders may have a stronger drive, be better informed and have a wider perspective than many others in the team, we don't have a monopoly over motivation and values and therefore, over what our col-lective vision might be. This is why 'telling' people what the direction they must take is inappropriate, although there is a balance to be struck between providing direction and being directive. People quickly lose confidence if they feel too much at sea, so our role not only includes facilitating but also getting the discussion off the ground, offering sug-gestions and clarifying what we could and should do together.

There are a number of ways of clarifying what matters to people and this does not always have to be done formally. For example, by noticing what goes on and how people feel, we may develop a good understanding of what they care about. We may then feel able to put this into words and express a vision on behalf of the team and check whether it resonates with them.

A more collaborative method is to bring people together and facilitate a discussion. We can jointly clarify our collective vision and aims by creating the space and then asking such questions as:

- Why are we doing this?
- What's important to us? Are we doing this?
- What are our values?
- How would we *not* want to go about doing things?
- How well are we doing?
- Where are we wasting our energy? Or on the wrong path?
- What should we be doing that we are not doing now?

Participation is the key to ownership and through facilitation, our job is to make participation easier, especially for those who are inhibited or don't feel they have the skills to articulate what they think and feel.

For example, it can be helpful to use notepaper and ask people to individually write down keywords or phrases. A word cloud can then be formed from which thoughts can be clustered and areas of commonality and difference noted. There is more on facilitation in Chapter 9.

Translating what has been shared into a succinct vision needn't be the work of the leader and could, for example, be made fun and inclusive, such as through a competition.

Who should we ask to contribute? In primary care, the appropriate people will include the primary care team, but could also include patients. Possibly it could include other organisations who are affected by, or could affect our work, such as commissioning agencies, social services, volunteering groups and colleagues in secondary care. In newly-forming communities, sharing purpose and values may help us to develop meaningful relationships with people who could become important allies.

If purpose is about why we do what we do, then values tell us something important about *how* we wish to go about doing that. In health care, 'values' are likely to include such virtues as being trustworthy, compassionate and professional. Our values might also include what people value about each other such as 'being supportive'. We can check that these are genuinely our core values, rather than simply ones that suit the current environment, by asking ourselves, 'If I moved to another practice tomorrow, would any of these values change?'

What really matters, is that these values are genuine. As leaders, we should encourage people to be honest about what they value, rather than coming out with what they think they *should* be saying. There are no 'right' values and they don't need to be validated by anyone external to the group. The practical point is that if the values are not genuine then the vision, the source of our energy, will be weak.

In a related way, as well as the *team's* core purpose, people have a *personal* core purpose that we could identify and use to connect with their individual 'why'. This becomes useful to explore when we are concerned about individuals who are struggling with the flow of their own motivation and energy.

Examples of a practice vision

Here are two examples of vision. In both of them, the shared *purpose* of delivering medical care is either explicit or implied. However, can you also see how the practices have infused their shared purpose with their *values*?

> The Coaltown medical centre describe their vision as being 'to provide excellent care for our community with compassion in our hearts and kindness in our processes'.

They came up with this wording after a discussion that identified that access problems and overwork were affecting their core value of compassion, and that systems such as the website and phone lines were alienating people, who found them cold and unhelpful.

> The Ash Green practice stated their vision as: 'By treating each other as family, we will have patients, colleagues and students queuing up to join our practice'.

For Ash Green, their core values include a strong supportive team spirit and being a culture where everyone learns from each other.

These visions, different for each practice, remind them of what they're aiming at. For their teams, their visions are powerful sources of energy because they connect with their hearts as well as their heads. How do the phrases seem to you? They may resonate, or alternatively they may leave you cold. If the latter, this would not be unnatural and is a reminder that a useful vision is not written for outsiders but for those within the organisation, for whom it should have meaning.

Articulating the vision and making it memorable

Writing a vision that is short, snappy and memorable is not an easy task and becomes harder the more people that are involved. Hence, we may want to write the vision with a small group of representatives from the community.

The vision is intended to be aspirational and to encourage us to reach, which is why it is neither phrased as an easily achievable task nor as something unattainable and impossible. As well as being inspiring, useful visions are easily understood, broad enough so that they don't narrow down the possibilities and are easy to get across. Think of them as something you could put on a T-shirt. Beware, however, T-shirt slogans can get a bad name because if they are not followed up with action, they appear glib.

For a vision to have impact, it should be difficult but possible to attain. To assist this, we can formulate an *audacious goal* which is one that is possible, but will require confidence and courage and may take years to achieve.

Purpose and values bring the energy of inspiration and to this, the audacious goal adds the energy of courage and resolve. A famous example of such a goal is the NASA moon mission in the 1960s. The vision had been to explore space, but the goal to put a man on the moon by the end of the decade and return him safely to earth was compelling and helped this become reality. In doing so, it created many other spin-off benefits along the way that were unanticipated.

For the Ash Green practice, with its strong training culture, an audacious goal based on their vision might be: 'Within 10 years, to become a community healthcare education hub, training the whole care team and educating our patients'.

Beyond the goal, to make it memorable, the vision should be described in vivid ways. It can be helpful to think of images, as these are even better than words at connecting with our emotions and are also much easier to recall and remind people of.

For example, the Greener Practice group in Sheffield [2] came together with a vision of changing the way health professionals behave so that they actively protect the environment as part of their role. The following image helped to encapsulate this synergy:

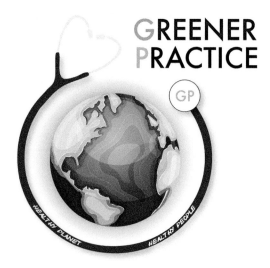

Combining vision, aims and strategy to set direction

At the start of the chapter, we stated that vision, aims and strategy help us to set direction.

However, they don't always have to be clarified in this sequence. Sometimes, having an aim (e.g. to use patient smartphone apps to improve remote diabetic management) may clarify the vision (to empower self-management and reduce dependency on GP clinics).

Beyond having a vision to connect them to, when formulating our aims, we need to check that they are appropriate and optimal. External sources can help, such as the diagram shown in the introduction to Section 5 that describes six dimensions of health care quality. We can use such a table to help us improve our aims.

In Chapter 23, we will explore in depth how to create an 'Aim Statement' for an improvement project and how to implement this using the model for improvement.

In setting direction, our *vision* tells us something about 'why' our action matters and our *aims* say more about 'what' we will do. We can then become more specific by developing our *strategy*, which guides 'how' we want to achieve our aims.

To draw a parallel, if the aim is to get from Sheffield to Stockport then our strategies are our broad options: we could go by train, car, or go on a hike across the Peak District. Once we've decided on a strategy, say going by rail, we can then develop more detailed objectives by asking: which stations are we using? how do we get to the station? what are the train times? and so on.

Back to practice life, where although there are many strategies, it can be helpful to think about different types that these fall into. This can broaden our thinking and increase our possibilities. Here is an example, illustrated further in the table below.

The Coaltown medical centre was concerned about depression and loneliness in young people and set the aim: 'To improve our community mental health service for teenagers and young adults'. Using a table of strategic options, it came up with the following possibilities.

AIM: TO IMPROVE OUR COMMUNITY MENTAL HEALTH SERVICE FOR YOUNG PEOPLE

TYPE OF STRATEGY	EXAMPLE
Provide information, enhance skills	Communicate better with young people, for example, talks in schools, information in different local languages
Enhance services and support	Improve our GP expertise, consider community psychiatrist in outreach clinic
Improve access, reduce barriers	Improve timings of clinics, consider telephone consultations
Motivate	Motivate parents and peers to recognise depression and refer for help
Change the policies or rules	Allow children to come without the parent's consent

It can be tempting to think of strategy as 'long-term planning', but perhaps that would be a mistake. As an organisation, we need to be agile and adaptable and it's helpful to think of strategy not as a way of keeping us resolutely on the rails, but as something that can be modified, perhaps like a steering wheel that can be turned when a change of direction is needed.

Let's summarise what we have learned in this chapter. We've used examples from the fictional Coaltown medical centre and in the table below, we bring together their vision, aim and strategy to show how these give the practice a clear, strong, and appropriate sense of direction.

CLARIFYING VISION AND DIRECTION AT THE COALTOWN MEDICAL CENTRE

WHAT WE DID	LEADER'S COMMENTS
Develop a vision: 'To provide excellent care for our community with compassion in our hearts and kindness in our processes'.	Initially, people were sceptical that developing a vision would be little more than ticking a managerial box. The hardest part was making sure that people were heard, especially the quiet ones and those who didn't have English as a first language. Also, people weren't sure how relevant this was or how it would make their lives easier. In reality, everyone had quite strong opinions and feelings and we all felt it was important to make them heard. The discussion brought out something important about our team which was that compassion and not letting the systems get in the way of the people, was what people most cared about and were concerned over. They wanted their work to connect to this, which they felt it didn't always.
Clarify an aim: 'To improve our community mental health service for young people'.	We work with a local school and from the children and teachers, we became aware of the significant mental health issues that young people had and how relatively little we were doing to address them. This tied in with our vision to provide compassionate care. When we considered the dimensions of quality, we could see that our treatment of young people was not *equitable* compared to other groups. This would be the area of quality that would be targeted by this aim.

(Continued)

CLARIFYING VISION AND DIRECTION AT THE COALTOWN MEDICAL CENTRE

WHAT WE DID	LEADER'S COMMENTS
Implement a strategy: 1 Improve access, reduce barriers by improving the timings of clinics and considering telephone consultations. 2 Change the policies or rules by allowing children to come without the parent's consent.	In line with our vision and aim, we identified a couple of strategies which not only addressed the aim, but did so in ways that allowed the processes and systems to be caring, rather than obstructive. I found the vision statement helpful in keeping us on track with developing appropriate strategies. Also, because I tried to find out what individuals were driven by, I was able to negotiate tasks that connected to their natural drives, which really helped to keep energy and motivation high.
Connecting people to the vision: Using the vision, aims and strategy as a tool.	I was also able to use the vision and aim to show as we went along that the work we were doing was clearly addressing what we had said was important. This helped to maintain momentum and morale and also helped to share responsibility. For example, I said in a group email 'A big "thank you" to Julia who gave up her lunch break to talk to a depressed schoolchild by phone today. We're all trying to give our young people better access to our care and Julia's generous action helped a vulnerable child at a critical time'.

We've seen one way of presenting our aims and strategy. There are other ways too, and in Chapter 23 we describe how to create a 'driver diagram' that lays out the aim and strategy as a 'plan on a page'.

Finally, a reminder not to frighten the horses. Setting direction and conveying enthusiasm transmits energy which some people feel is motivating but others experiences as pressure that makes them feel anxious, or even overwhelmed. Because of the positive nature of the message, they might find it impossible to express their anxiety, so the onus is on us as leaders to be sensitive, alert and tailor the way we communicate accordingly.

Over the stile

In primary care, our work can be so reactive that there seems little time to do much more than firefighting. 'Setting direction' seems like a luxury, but good leaders recognise its importance and make time for it. We've seen in this chapter that it's perfectly feasible and can be invaluable in giving the team a sense of purpose and control. If our colleagues do not feel that the ship is rudderless and lacking direction, confidence is maintained. Energy is therefore dissipated in anxiety, but can be applied to oars pulled by a (mostly) willing crew.

Once we've agreed where we are headed and are ready to put in the effort, we then need fresh ideas to help us adapt and evolve. People are potentially very creative in seeing things differently and coming up with ideas, but how do we help them make use of that potential? We will consider that aspect of our leadership as we move on to the next chapter.

References

1. Sinek, S. How great leaders inspire action. www.ted.com/talks/simon_sinek_how_great_leaders_inspire_action. Accessed 19 November 2019.
2. Greener Practice Group Sheffield. Healthy Planet Healthy People. www.greener-practice.co.uk/. Accessed 20 January 2020.

18

Help the team to get more, and better, ideas

In this chapter, we will explore these questions:

- What holds people back and how can we encourage them to contribute?
- What encourages conformity (groupthink) and how could we counter this?
- What techniques can we use to help people use their own perspective and also to use ones that they may not have thought of?

As we've established, leaders don't necessarily have the best ideas and therefore, the legitimacy to have their ideas preferred over those of others. In Chapter 5, we touched on why the differences between us are so important to the team and here we discuss how to engage those differences to get better ingredients for making changes, that is, better ideas on the issues, options and actions that we should consider. Of course, the process of generating ideas does not occur in a vacuum. The context, particularly, the nature of the problem, is discussed in detail in Section 5. It is this context that catalyses the creative thinking that we explore here.

Encouraging people to contribute

If we want to engage differences, we have to recruit people who *are* different and are not just images of ourselves or each other. Tools such as personality and role inventories are used in some organisations to identify what we are lacking.

It's quite likely that our existing teams are already diverse, but do we harness this? Because we are different, we are able to generate different ideas between us, in other words to be creative. Creativity therefore isn't a matter of having particular skills so much as having the confidence to value what is within each of us and then having the opportunity to use it. Our task as leaders is to facilitate that.

To encourage people to open up, we create a safe environment where ideas are welcomed. We avoid leading the discussions, as this sets the tone for what is acceptable or preferred. This takes discipline as people may look to us to do exactly that. Instead, we help people to voice ideas and reinforce this behaviour by handling their ideas respectfully.

Even while taking care not to be too controlling, we still need to give direction. This is because people are bolder and have more and better suggestions when they are clearer about the question, issue or task.

Here are some ways forward:

- Make contributing easy; for example, a small Post-it note is not as intimidating as a blank sheet of A4 paper.
- Think of ideas as gifts.
- Suspend judgement. Be very careful with body language and try not to look unhappy. With some people, looking thoughtful can be misinterpreted as being concerned, so we may have to warn colleagues not to misread us.
- More obviously we should not be dismissive or categorise ideas as being 'bad'; after all, many great changes have arisen from ideas that were originally ridiculed or dismissed.
- Encourage people to keep opening up and build on their ideas by avoid saying 'yes, but', and instead saying 'yes, and?'.
- Act on ideas and remind people of our history of doing so; people contribute more when they know it leads to something and makes a difference.
- Show the team, perhaps by acknowledging the contributions, that they have ownership. Remember that colleagues don't just support, but actually fight for what they have helped to create.

It is helpful to remember that stepping back, not taking the credit and being generous are really important facilitators in this context. We get something important from this too, because encouraging the contribution of others is a significant way of nurturing our humility.

Discouraging people from thinking the same

A lack of disagreement or alternative viewpoints is known to lead to poor decisions because an insufficient range of information to inform decisions is generated and analysed. This can happen particularly when there is a strong persuasive or controlling group leader, who might narrow the discussion.

Conformity and groupthink (1) have their origin in a number of places, which include:

- *Peer pressure* to conform to what the group is thinking, for example, 'If you feel like we are going in the wrong direction, you can always work on something else or join a different team'.
- *Stereotyping:* 'well, the receptionists are bound to disagree because they're always saying they can't take any more on'.
- *No one speaks against.* This can give the illusion of unanimity.
- *Self-censoring:* 'If everyone else is in agreement, then my thoughts must be wrong'.

  People who are a 'fresh pair of eyes' have valuable ideas because they are less blinkered. However, because they are new to the community, they are especially likely to self-censor.

Groupthink is less likely to happen if we watch out for these behaviours and positively encourage people to open up. In addition, we can make sure as leaders that we encourage (but don't necessarily support) opposing views, encourage people to explore alternatives and get them to comment on the risks of any course of action and how much they think these risks matter.

Facilitating people to think differently

In addition to the background work described earlier, there are techniques that can help the group think more widely and more deeply. Here are a few that are worth researching further and trying out.

Brainstorming: This is widely used to encourage people to open up in a group setting. There are rules to encourage more contribution, such as avoiding criticism and postponing judgement.

Brainwriting: This is a good alternative or a complement to brainstorming, and it often yields more ideas in less time than traditional group brainstorming.

People initially work independently, writing their thoughts for example on post-it notes, which are then passed on to another participant who can add thoughts triggered by the earlier ones and so on round the group. This carries on for about 15 minutes and the results are then collated. The technique allows everyone to have a voice, not just the noisy or more powerful ones, so no one is intimidated by the *people*.

Because it feels safer, more radical ideas can also be suggested than when they have to be shouted out loud. Because it's private and on a Post-it note, everyone can contribute, so no one feels intimidated by the *task*.

Starbursting is an alternative approach in which a six-pointed star is drawn on a large sheet of paper and the following words are put on the points: Why, What, When, How, Who and Where.

The name of the idea, problem or task is written in the centre of the star, and there is then a brainstorming/brainwriting session using each point as a prompt.

SCAMPER (2) is another technique that uses prompts. In this, each letter stands for a mental process we can apply to a budding idea. The letters stand for:

- Substitute
- Combine
- Adapt
- Magnify/Modify/Minimize
- Put to other uses
- Eliminate
- Reverse/Rearrange

In this technique, we are not just relying on the diversity of how people think in order to generate ideas, but are also prompting different ways of thinking about a problem. Following is an example of how it could be used.

The problem: A lot of our GP workload comes from musculoskeletal problems, especially back pain. How could we manage this differently?

TECHNIQUE	IDEA
Substitute	Instead of patients being directed to the doctor, could the GP be **substituted** by another practitioner such as a physiotherapist to perform the assessment?
Combine	If the physio worked alongside the GPs, the patient could be assessed and passed across for investigation if necessary, at the same visit. In this way, the skills of both professionals could be **combined**.
Adapt	Could we **adapt** using new technology? Could patients do their own triage using an online assessment?
Magnify/Modify/Minimize	Could we **modify** our current assessment approach, for example, develop a template that prompted all the red and yellow clinical flags to aid decision making? This could speed up assessment and make it more consistent between different practitioners (including doctors/non-doctors) and safer overall.
Put to other uses	Could we **put GPs to other uses** and employ a musculoskeletal practitioner who would take over the medical assessment and be able to prescribe?
Eliminate	Could we **eliminate** some of the workload through health education, teaching people about methods of preventing back problems through posture, activity, back strengthening and stretching exercises?
Reverse/Rearrange	Instead of patients coming to doctors for assessment and then being sent for investigation, could we **reverse** this? They could be triaged, investigated and then sent to a doctor with the results of tests.

Although this technique is not intuitive, it can lead to ideas we may not have otherwise thought of. As with all the techniques discussed here, this is simply a tool to be experimented with individually and in combination with others.

Six Hats is an idea from Edward de Bono, the father of lateral thinking (3). Each coloured hat is a different perspective or attitude. It's fun as well as creative especially if people really inhabit the role, for example by *wearing* the different coloured hats. It can be used by groups of people or by individuals to see the issue from a different perspective and it gives them permission to play 'devil's advocate'. In addition, a problem can also be worked through by using the hats in a recommended sequence, which brings additional insights.

It's very hard for us as individuals to 'be someone else', to truly use the perspective of someone who sees the world in a different way. Hence, getting people to wear each hat in turn is great for problem-solving but also for broadening our awareness of diversity, improving our mutual understanding and reducing unnecessary conflict.

In addition to these examples, there are specific tools that we can use as part of the quality improvement process to analyse the workplace. With this information, we can generate further problem-solving ideas and these tools are discussed in depth in Chapter 22.

Over the stile

We have seen in this chapter that the creativity of our colleagues comes from their differences. We've discussed how to give them the confidence to use their differences in generating ideas. This process helps people to value each other but also illuminates the *divergence* between us.

In the next chapter, we will focus on *convergence*. Specifically, how do we bring people who come from different positions, sufficiently together so that they can develop and agree on proposals for change?

References

1. Janis, I.L. (1982). *Groupthink: Psychological Studies of Policy Decisions and Fiascoes.* Boston: Houghton Mifflin. ISBN: 0-395-31704-5.
2. Eberele, R.S. (2008). *Creative Games and Activities for Imagination Development.* Waco, TX: Prufrock Press Inc. ISBN-13: 987-1-59363-346-7.
3. de Bono, E. Six thinking hats. www.debonogroup.com/six_thinking_hats.php. Accessed 27 January 2020.

19

Create buy-in and build consensus

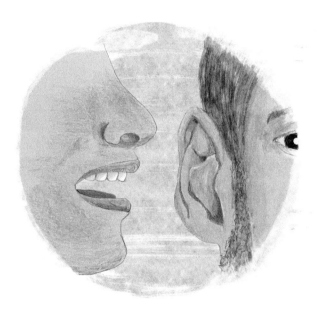

- What is persuasion and why is it necessary?
- How do we make our case persuasive to people with different perspectives?
- How do we get agreement when people start from different positions?
- What is the difference between consensus and compromise?

Persuasion

Persuasion is used at various times in the change process, including when we argue the need for change, promote one idea or option over another or persuade people to commit their effort to a course of action. Here, we will focus on how people commit to the need for change and commit to taking an active role in making improvements.

As we've noted before, the minute we use our authority to insist on compliance, we scupper our chance to connect. This is because we fail to respect the powerful intrinsic motivation that our colleagues possess which can be enlisted but cannot be commanded.

This is where using persuasion becomes important. Persuasion is not manipulation or coercing people to do something that is not in their interest. It is the art of encouraging people through reasoning and argument, to believe in something or commit to something that is in our joint interest.

Connecting the need for change to our shared vision is an important first step for reasons that we discussed in Chapter 17. Indeed as leaders, where the change we are being asked to take on is *not* compatible with our purpose or interests, we may have to stand up on behalf of our colleagues and resist the pressure to comply.

Persuading people is not just about pitching to them. It is a process rather than an event and is based on something deeper, which is that to move forward, both leaders and the rest of the team have to understand each other's positions and be prepared to shift to find common ground. We sometimes call this buying-in or aligning ourselves with each other. We should acknowledge that despite persuasion and consensus-building, it isn't always possible for leaders and their community to align. There will be instances where one party will need to go with the will of the other. Such sacrifices are not common but are noted by the other parties and can enhance trust.

Using a series of questions, let's now consider the process of persuasion in more detail from the viewpoint of the leader, or indeed anyone doing the persuading.

Do I have a helpful attitude?

Most importantly, we need to be *seen* to be open-minded. We should be careful about being dogmatic and should show through our language and behaviour that we are prepared to think again about our position.

This behaviour will also encourage, if not guarantee, greater flexibility in those we are conversing with.

Who could be affected by the change and what is their position?

As part of the process of persuasion, especially in advance of any presentation that we might make to others, it's really important that we seek out the people who will be significantly impacted by the change, listen carefully to their thoughts and concerns and find out how they feel emotionally.

What are their priorities? If they are resistant, where might the barriers lie and what might they be afraid of losing? In terms of loss, this could include concerns over job security and workload, but could also include important but less tangible things like autonomy, status, influence and well-being.

How could I help them to move to a new position?

Seeking people out, as described above, is likely to lead to difficult conversations. If we talk with them, we may be credited for showing that we care, although that's not guaranteed. What's more certain is that if we don't talk, it will be held against us and getting people on board will become all the more difficult down the line.

We also need to be clear in our minds about *why* the change is needed and be able to explain the benefits of taking action and the risks of *not* doing so.

If as a result of this dialogue people end up caring, they may also end up committing.

How can I make the case compellingly?

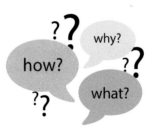

Perhaps we could start with how *not* to do it. Persuasion is not about a hard sell. It's not about being tough and avoiding concessions or thinking that people will be bowled over by a great argument or presentation. A rational case is important, but it's only one part of the equation.

Persuasion is also not a one-off effort, like a presentation, speech or meeting. It's a longer process because it's about developing an on-going relationship.

Let's now focus on an important part of the process of persuasion, which is our pitch. This may be planned or opportunistic, but in both cases, people need to be helped to appreciate that we have a shared problem, that there is a credible way forward and that their contribution matters.

It is worth developing what is known as an 'elevator pitch', meaning something that can be used opportunistically and said quickly, as if we were in a lift between the floors of a building. This should be energising, get to the nub of the matter and leave the listener interested to know more. However, for a planned meeting or event, we have the time to do a much more informed pitch, and here are some key features that help us to make that more compelling:

- **Preparation** is vital and in addition to what we have discussed earlier, we might check out the mood of those who will be there, where and with whom the blocks might lie and how our proposal might go down. This we do by talking to trusted colleagues beforehand.

- **Timing** matters and we should choose an optimal time, such as when there isn't another urgent priority, when resources are available or when the issue has also become important to other people who could become potential allies.

- **Credibility** shouldn't be taken for granted. People will be asking themselves: 'Can I believe this person?' and 'What are the implications for me?'. Usually, our credibility will already be established in the practice because people know us well. If not, then we might have to find other ways of demonstrating our credibility, for example, from our qualifications, experience, achievements or from our behaviour, such as being seen to be open and not rigid.

- **Reaching out** is important. We should frame the proposal in a way that shows we understand and empathise with how people feel. We may also wish to show how the proposal has been (or could be) modified to take account of their concerns.

- **Connecting to the 'Why'.** We shouldn't forget to describe the proposal in ways that also connect with people emotionally and help them to feel that this *matters* to them and to the team. Stories and images are powerful ways of getting this across. For instance, let's suppose we were proposing a new clinic for children with learning disabilities. We might say: 'As you know John, our previous practice manager who did so much for the practice has a disabled child, who when she was young received very little help from her own practice. Times have changed and we, in this practice, can do much better, so let's set up a new clinic that would make John proud'.

- **Be rational.** To balance our appeal to the emotions, we need to show that we are also clear-headed. We can do this partly by having a rational case, but also by using data, which needs to be powerful, sparse, clear and to the point. Data in the form of tables, graphs and so on is disproportionately powerful and is often underused.

- *Use people's preferences.* We all have our preferred way of describing and explaining, which reflects the way we see the world. It's really helpful to remember that different people are biased to listen out for different things:
  - Some want to know *why* this is important and why they should care. Connecting with feelings and motivation will attract their attention.
  - Others want to know *what* the reasoning is and the evidence that underpins it. Using reasoning and logic will have them listening closely.
  - The third group don't care about either of these so much as the practical implications of *how* we are going to go about it. Using practical illustrations of what we need to do next to implement the idea, will bring them to life.
- We will have our own natural style which may focus on one of these perspectives, but we can become more persuasive by making sure that we cover *all* these perspectives in our presentation.
- We can also become more persuasive if we learn to engage people in a variety of ways including addressing their fears, connecting with what we know they are motivated by or by being energising or light-hearted as well as serious.
- During the meeting, we should be sensitive to the emotions in the room and be prepared to adjust and respond to these, rather than slavishly follow a plan.
- Reputations are quickly tarnished through failing to deliver, so to manage expectations it can be helpful to under-promise on those expectations with the intention of over-delivering on the task.
- Relationships matter more than positions and all victories and losses are only temporary. Therefore, whether the important decision went for or against us, we should follow up by going to those who were on the opposite side of the debate to show that we can take 'winning or losing', well. If we are seen not to gloat if we succeed, or to have hard feelings if we don't, we can maintain relationships and trust for the debates that the future will hold.

How do we move to a position that we can jointly commit to?

No one likes a fait accompli and because our intention is not to dictate but to negotiate a way forward, we need to reflect this in our language. By asking our colleagues for their help and by being flexible, people are much more likely to engage. We might say things like 'What if?', 'I need your help' or 'Would it be helpful if...?'.

If a shared position is not yet clear, we could invite those involved to discuss and even debate the merits of the proposal, offering honest feedback and suggesting alternatives. As an example of alternatives and how these could be structured to facilitate debate, look at the options appraisal in the managing change section of Chapter 24. This has the helpful effect of shifting the issue from conflict-resolution into a problem-solving context.

We could also consult more widely or find out if a coalition is possible, teaming up with other people for whom this problem is also an issue. It's harder for colleagues to stand in the way if they recognise that the problem affects communities beyond those who have come with a proposal.

Case example

Peter, a GP partner, was keen to employ a physician's associate as there was a shortage of doctors. The practice was concerned about the cost, but Peter was able to show that the nurses had similar concerns about practice nurse recruitment and that a physician's associate would help both teams. This softened his colleagues' attitudes.

Ultimately, we should be genuinely willing to consider adjusting our position, not out of tokenism but because common ground is a starting point, not an endpoint. The sooner we can start working together on the proposal, the sooner we will all move forwards and achieve something worthwhile.

This encourages people to make small initial commitments in the knowledge that doing so doesn't signify fully signed-up acceptance but indicates pragmatism and a willingness to find a way forward. As leaders, we may have to take a lead in modelling this.

To paraphrase Mario Cuomo, 'We persuade through poetry but take action through prose', meaning that persuasion is subtle and indirect like poetry and prepares us for the more down-to-earth work of undertaking tasks.

Facilitating consensus, avoiding compromise

We have considered how we can try to get people to commit to change, but there will come a point when options will be generated and fought over.

Sometimes, even though teams may generate options, the choice of which to select may not be theirs to make. As we discussed in Chapter 13, the ground rules for a task-based team should include ones on how decisions are made. These should have been clarified at the outset in order to prevent expectations being falsely raised.

More usually however, the group has a strong part to play in deciding how to move forward. This will need discussion in which we, as leaders, will play a part. Our role is to discover, not dictate, what we collectively think is possible and what we can jointly endorse. Let's compare and contrast the roles that compromise and consensus have to play in achieving this.

Compromise is commonplace, but is potentially unhelpful because it doesn't facilitate discovery, but starts from the end and works backwards. Characteristically with the process of compromise, people enter dialogue with pre-formed positions on what they believe would be acceptable to *them*. Such positions are unlikely to be acceptable to the whole group at the outset, because there has not yet been opportunity for discussion and disclosure. There will therefore be disagreement and because of this, there has to be an attempt to find common ground.

If compromise is used to find common ground, those involved:

- Give away something that they feel is essential,
- In order to get something from others, and
- In the hope that there will be a future agreement in which they win back some of what they have given up under pressure.

As we can see, compromise makes use of manipulation and control, which is why it may be unhelpful. So, what of consensus, which is an alternative way of finding an area of agreement?

Consensus is different and the derivation of the word, which is 'feeling together', is enlightening. People come into the process with more open minds and with questions rather than positions. The ensuing discussion takes those involved on a journey of discovering what others think, feel, hold dear, worry about or believe is possible and less possible.

As leaders, we can facilitate this process and it is helpful for us to consider why people disagree. To keep it simple, here are three major reasons and for each, some interventions and phrases that we might use to clarify where people stand and to help them reach consensus.

HELPING THE TEAM TO REACH CONSENSUS

WHY DO PEOPLE DISAGREE?	HOW COULD WE HELP?
They are not hearing each other	• Get each party to listen one-by-one to each other • Structure the discussion so everyone can speak and be heard ('We'll go round so that everyone can put their point of view') • Encourage people to respect strong opinions and not squash them • Depersonalise the discussion so that ideas are not too strongly linked with the author *(Continued)*

HELPING THE TEAM TO REACH CONSENSUS

WHY DO PEOPLE DISAGREE?	HOW COULD WE HELP?
	• Where do people stand? • Encourage people to be open not only about what they think, but what they feel, and make sure there are no reprisals for doing this ('We need to be honest with each other and respect each other's opinions') • Summarise and check for understanding
They have different values and experiences and interpret what they hear, differently	• Help the group to discuss the proposal, its pros and cons and how it might impact upon them. In particular, because people fear loss rather than change, find out what those in disagreement feel they might lose if that option was selected • Clarify what people agree about • Confirm the sources of disagreement • Encourage people to use reasoning ('Can you explain what makes you feel/think that way?', 'What do you see are the implications of doing that?') • Through the questions asked, identify any invalid assumptions and discard them • Help to clarify the options so that they can be compared fairly with each other ('What are the choices here and the pros and cons of each?') • Explain that consensus is not about getting all that *you* want, but coming up with an agreement that *everyone* can accept
It is due to external factors, like interpersonal conflict	• Don't attempt to resolve the issue in the group session • Meet the people concerned privately to discuss a way forward, which might include going to a higher authority or using an intermediary to help them resolve conflicts

When necessary, if agreement can't be reached through discussion, we can use techniques such as voting not to make the decision, but to assist the discussion process. For example, we can use voting to whittle down the options.

The consensus when it is reached, may be for something less ambitious than some would have wished. This is to be expected, but because the consensus is a starting point for progress, not the finishing line, we can be reassured that we have a solid foundation on which to build.

Because consensus comes from a deep place which probes what people are fearful of losing, the process becomes much more fluent and effective when people trust each other. As leaders, we could help the group to build trust (if we have the opportunity) through activities such as socialising.

As the discussion proceeds, the common ground or consensus grows large enough for the group to act upon. However, compromise may still have a place. For example, if consensus is not found to be possible for everyone, those unpersuaded might compromise to allow things to proceed.

As leaders, we need to remember that those who have compromised will not be signed up and may not only be unhappy but also may work against progress, either by not contributing or worse still through sabotage. These people need to be kept on side and supported in future discussions. They are not enemies to be marginalised but are colleagues whose willingness to compromise so as not to block progress should be appreciated, perhaps publicly.

Over the stile

We've seen the importance of getting people on board and helping them to find common ground from which they can move forwards. Facilitating this process isn't easy, even with the willingness and patience to do so.

It often takes place piecemeal in informal settings, but sometimes a more structured approach is required. In the next chapter, we explore how effective chairs help to build consensus in more formal meetings.

20

Chair effectively

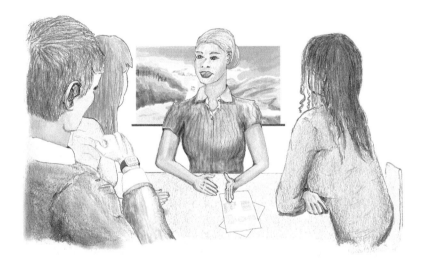

In this chapter, we will explore these questions:

- What skills and attitudes are important in the role?
- How could our feel for people's attitudes and behaviour help us to chair well?
- How could we recognise and manage difficult behaviour?

Meetings are frequent, and usually they are relatively informal and require a degree of facilitation rather than needing a chair. However, in situations when the issues are more significant, the stakes are higher and more people are involved, chairing can be invaluable. Meetings that have a chair are usually formal, with an agenda-led discussion.

We will not discuss formal meeting rules here, which might include checking previous minutes for accuracy and following up on action points, but instead will focus on the chair's role and skills in facilitating the discussion.

Who should be chair?

Being chair is not just a title or position but also a skill. Therefore, even though we may be a leader in the group, it doesn't necessarily mean that we will be the best person to chair the meeting. This is especially the case if we need to play a major part in the discussion, because the role of the chair is to facilitate the group's discussion rather than to have a strong influence over the content or outcomes of that dialogue.

What are the skills and attitudes involved?

Here is a brief overview of what the chair needs to do in the meeting:

- Clarify the aims and objectives of the discussion
- Ensure the meeting flows smoothly by involving all members present
- Exercise control by not permitting one or two people to dominate the meeting
- Avoid dominating as chair or inappropriately closing down discussion
- The chair should also summarise during meetings to:
  - Indicate progress, or lack of
  - Refocus discussion that has wandered off the point
  - Conclude one point and lead on to the next
  - Highlight important points
  - Assist the secretary if necessary
  - Clarify any misunderstanding
- Ensure that decisions are made and not put off
- Ensure that decisions are representative of the views expressed
- Arrange appropriate follow-up

The attitudes and skills involved are very similar to those of leadership itself, because these meetings are a microcosm of the process of change, condensed to a small space and a short period in time. Therefore as you read this chapter, imagine how you might apply the insights you gain here, to become more effective leaders as well as better chairs.

The shape of chairing

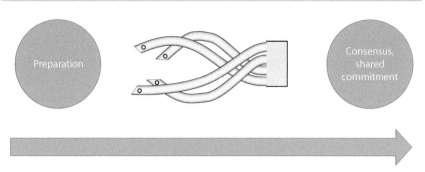

Preparation

Consensus, shared commitment

Let's imagine chairing as a process, rather than as an event. To visualise this, we will give it the shape shown in the diagram which illustrates some important phases of chairing. Preparation is clearly important, and this is followed by the meeting itself in which we become aware of four strands of behaviour, which we seek to bring together in some form of consensus. The consensus may not be to go ahead with a proposal, it may be quite the opposite, but our task is not to presume the outcome but to facilitate it so that people agree on the next steps forward.

What are these phases and how can we navigate them?

Preparation

This involves establishing the agenda, which we will share with all partici-pants before the meeting. As an example let's consider an agenda item that needs discussion, rather than just presentation. We will need to find out who is attending and get the agenda item clarified so that we understand what needs to be discussed, why it has been put forward and what decision is required from the group. This is likely to involve a conversation with the proposer that helps to refine the initial proposal, so that it can be discussed more effectively and not go off on a number of tangents that could distract the discussion and lead to an unsatisfactory meeting.

Because our role is to facilitate the discussion, we need to understand before the meeting the main concerns that people might have, the areas of contention and where the bear traps might lie that could ensnare the discussion. This involves contacting and where necessary seeing people, especially if they are unfamiliar to us, and taking soundings on what mat-ters to whom.

In the meeting: the four strands

Being chair is a trusted position and our attitude is very important and helps to set the tone for the meeting. In our own minds, our focus is on the process and outcomes and not so much on the individuals and their personalities. This helps us to be more objective and to avoid being overly biased for or against particular people. We need to try our best to behave as an 'honest broker' and to be seen as being impartial and fair-minded.

If we want the group to have a genuine discussion rather than just stating dogmatic positions, we need to encourage them to be open-minded and to feel able to contribute. Therefore, despite temptation or provocation, we need to model this by remaining open-minded ourselves, encouraging mutual respect and ensuring everyone has their voice. There will also be someone keeping a record, and we can assist them to make sure that this record is a fair and useful representation of what transpires.

Being chair is hard work, mainly because it requires intense concentration to notice, then to interpret not only what people are saying but also how they are feeling, as expressed through their non-verbal communication. This requires great communication skills and in particular, a high degree of emotional awareness.

Let's take this further. At a superficial level, we need to keep the meeting on track and prevent unhelpful behaviour from diverting its main purpose. A few pointers about this are given later. However, at a deeper level we need to learn to *read the room* and get a feel for how supportive and committed people are to the proposal and the process.

To clarify, being supportive in this context means that people are prepared to see the proposal go through. Being committed means that people are also willing to assist the implementation of the proposal. These two dimensions are deep features. Have you been aware of them in meetings that you have attended?

As shown in the following table, we can think of these in terms of four strands. They represent four responses rather than four types of people, because each of us can move between the four as the discussion progresses. Our aim as chair is to notice these responses and guide people towards a shared position, where this is possible. In the table below are some thoughts on how we might interpret what we notice and based on this, how we might help.

THE 'FOUR STRANDS' OF RESPONSE TO THE DISCUSSION	OUR THOUGHTS AND EXAMPLES OF HOW WE MIGHT HELP
Supportive of the proposal, but not committed to it	• It may be good that they are supportive and therefore less likely to stand in the way. However, we shouldn't assume that support indicates a lack of concern. Perhaps they do not understand the issues, which may need to be clarified? • We **need to check** whether there are any aspects that they have strong views about and whether, once they understand the proposal, they are still in support.
Supportive of the proposal and committed	• These people are clearly allies of the proposal. We might invite them to use their positivity to come up with options for a way forward. Their expectations will be high, so we need to manage these to avoid people becoming disappointed. We could therefore involve allies of the proposal in setting *feasible objectives.*
Critical of the proposal but committed	• We might think of these people as being critical friends. Criticism and resistance are really important, because they stop the organisation from walking off the cliff edge through being unrealistic or too carried away with excitement. • We might first check that their judgement is credible and then ask ourselves: *do they have a point?* Have they seen something that others haven't noticed? *How would they modify the proposal* to a more acceptable position? Or what steps should we take to establish whether their concerns are justified?
Critical of the proposal and not committed	• This can be the toughest group. Might they be in denial? Again, clarification of the proposal is important and in particular, what problem the proposal is addressing and *why* it is needed. • *What are their main concerns?* People resist loss rather than change, so what do they fear losing? What would they most like to preserve (and is there some way that this can be accommodated)? What do they feel would make this issue important to them?

As we can see from the table, there are no good or bad strands of response, as each of these brings a different perspective that is helpful to the process. For example:

- What we might otherwise call dissent or negativity can actually help to keep us on track and bring up considerations that are important to all of us,
- Critics can help us to be wise *before* the event,
- Positivity brings positive energy that keeps us upbeat, but may blinker us or make us set objectives that are unrealistic.

From the comments in the table, we can see that for each strand there are potentially constructive responses from the chair that keep people involved and hopefully stop them becoming dominant or marginalised. When people see, through the chair's behaviour, that they are respected enough to be kept involved, they may become less likely to disrupt the process, unless of course their motives are suspect or devious. Let's move on to consider this.

Managing difficult behaviour

People may have their own agenda, different degrees of commitment to the process and based on these, different forms of behaviour. They may behave with integrity, but they may not and may become mischievous or disruptive.

Generally, we are not dealing with bad people. People join the NHS with good intentions and to make things better for patients, but sometimes they lose their way. When people behave badly, rather than being because they are wicked, it may be that they are losing their moral courage. Chairing is a form of leadership, and as chairs we can help people by being open, honest and clear about the need to behave with integrity, and to help each other.

Despite all this, there are people who will use meetings to score points and to further their own agenda. If we are aware of this, we can develop a range of techniques to help us manage any behaviour that does not respect people or the purpose of the meeting. Ethically, we can justify this on the basis of doing our best for the group. In so doing, it's possible we can also help the individuals concerned to modify their behaviour and become more useful members of the group. For example, by recognising their helpful contributions or their attempts to be more flexible.

In the next section, we give some direct quotes from a chair with much experience in these high-stakes environments (Mr Ian Hammond, former NHS Trust Chief Executive, personal communication, June 4, 2019).

You may or may not resonate with these, but the suggestions raised will help you to reflect on how you have previously responded in these situations and how you might do so in the future.

General guidance

The following points illustrate useful attitudes and approaches that we might use as chair:

- Agree the ground rules for behaviour
- Be courteous, respectful and – if you can – charming; this will win over waverers
- Be nice to everyone; you never know when you might need them
- Focus on the desired outcome, not the process
- Be prepared – have your frequently asked questions (FAQ) script ready
- Be as honest as you can, including telling people when you don't know and when you can't say
- Try to judge on the basis of objective facts not on whether you like or dislike an individual
- Give the impression you know less than you actually do
- Avoid getting too close to anyone; for every friend you make you will attract their enemies and you will be seen as partisan
- Try to identify good practice – even if it is only relative
- Remain calm, however angry you feel – this puts the aggressor on the back foot
- Bullies are basically cowards so bite back … gently
- Identify why it is in their own interest to behave
- Wherever possible, avoid apologising. For example, use 'And your point is?'
- Avoid anything you would be embarrassed about
- Define your availability and stick to it because people invade; have other commitments to go to – including home and social

Specific guidance

In any walk of life, people are often the most challenging element. The following table shows a number of negative or unhelpful behaviours and suggestions on how we might manage them to keep the meeting on track.

TYPE OF PERSON/BEHAVIOUR	POSSIBLE RESPONSE
Disrespectful	Use adult-adult not parent-child
Rude	'There's no need to be rude'
Aggressive	Silence (and deep breathing)
Passive aggressive	'Is there a problem?'
Bullying	Stand firm – be assertive
Being bounced	Refuse to be suckered in –say no
Disengaged	Persistence (is there a problem?)
Lacking boundaries	Stick to boundaries
Disloyalty	Watch your back and gather evidence
Disobedient	They may have misunderstood
Untruthful	Tell the truth – and record it
Undermining	Make alliances and expose it
Don't deliver	Monitor and have a Plan B
Blabbermouth	Trace the source, then tackle it
'Forgetful'	Record your understanding
Chronic ill health	Be sympathetic – it is the NHS after all
Drug/alcohol dependence	Confidential chat – it will always be a wider problem

Over the stile

At the end of Section 4 of this book, we now have a better appreciation of how to value the differences between us enough to harness them, be more creative and through consensus-building and good facilitation, find common ground for moving forward.

The team are now ready to get down to the nuts and bolts of implementing change, and to do this they need not proceed in a haphazard way. There is a scientific approach that we can use that makes the most of our experience so that we can experiment, learn, adapt and improve. We could think of this as being trial and learning, rather than trial and error. The stile ahead beckons us to this terrain, which we will now explore in detail.

5

Our tools: Making things better

Section introduction

We've discussed *how* we come together with others to work effectively. We are now moving on to talk about *what* we might be working on and talk about specific techniques that will help us in the task.

Leading any part of the health service is a constant process of managing change. Some of this change is imposed upon our organisations by our contractors or our regulators. However, most of our day-to-day leadership interventions relate to finding better ways of doing things to improve the quality of our patient care, and the working lives of ourselves and our team members.

As leaders in healthcare, we are aiming to provide high quality care for the population we serve. So what does high quality healthcare look like? In 2001, the US Institute of Medicine created a framework for healthcare quality which helps to guide us when deciding what areas of our practice may benefit from improvement.

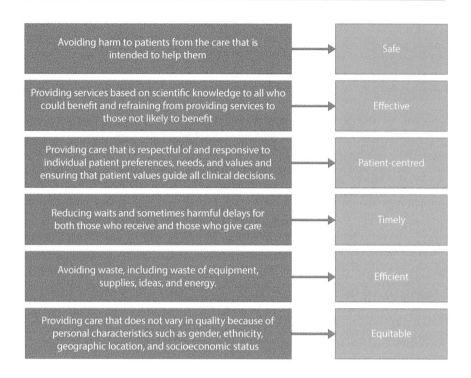

The six areas defined have become known as the 'Six domains of health-care quality'. They are noble aspirations and help to define *what* we are aiming to achieve, but not *how* we will achieve it.

The choices that we make when leading improvement will make a difference to both the success and the sustainability of what we do. And it is so easy to get it wrong. Just think of the times we have implemented something we thought was a good idea but had failed to really understand how it might impact on the team. How tempting it is to pay for a piece of software that 'promises' to manage all our patient recall for long-term condition reviews but which ends up making a mess of a system that had been evolving beautifully over many years. Do we fall in the trap of opting for the first idea rather than the best idea? Or take a lead from the loudest voice rather than the whole team?

Often making improvements doesn't require skilled leadership because it's straightforward. Just installing an automatic check-in screen or an automatic front door can make our practice more efficient and equitable.

Good leadership comes in when we need to tackle more complex challenges. This is when it is useful to make a distinction between 'improving quality' and 'quality improvement' (QI). QI has acquired a more specific meaning that includes employing a structured, systematic approach to improvement. It involves gaining a deeper understanding of the problem that needs to be fixed, and then testing out changes to see which makes the most difference, whilst paying constant attention to the experience of the users of the service and the engagement of teams who deliver the care.

Good QI involves testing out changes and seeing if they start to generate the difference we want to see. For us, this is what makes QI such an exciting area to lead, as it encourages all who work within a service to participate in improving care for patients, and also improving their working lives. As QI is a process of controlled experimentation with new ideas it is dynamic and inclusive. If it becomes 'built in' to our day-to-day work, it can also help to shift our practice culture and generate increased joy at work.

Learning QI skills is partly about trying out new tools, but it is also about a change in mindset. It's easy to become disheartened if we implement a change that hasn't worked. If we are genuine in our sense of 'testing out' new things, then we will be pleased to have learned what doesn't work, as much as what does work. It's the continuous learning that drives us toward our quality goal. As leaders we have a constant eye on both the task and the process, trying to bring people with us, keep them engaged and maintain our own motivation. A structured QI approach can help to do all of this as well as help to convince people who are sceptical. Experimentation and getting it wrong are appropriate and positive, rather than a risky threat to confidence.

Don Berwick (2013), former president of the US Institute of Healthcare Improvement chaired a review on improving the safety of patients in the English NHS. The published report, 'A Promise to Learn – A Commitment to Act', included the statement: *'The most important single change in the NHS in response to this report would be for it to become, more than ever before, a system devoted to continual learning and improvement of patient care, top to bottom and end to end'.*

In this section, we will be sharing our experience of QI in general practice, showing how to use established tools to support the various stages of the process. To help in navigating the chapter we divide up the QI process into stages:

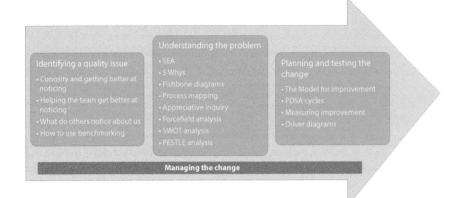

- *Identifying a quality issue* – How do we know what we need to improve?

- *Understanding the problem* – How do we broaden and deepen our understanding before rushing in with a fix?

- *Planning and testing the change* – How do we safely experiment and measure if we are on the right track?

- *Managing the change* – How do we understand and manage the human response to change?

This section is probably the most 'technical' of our book, and gives some very practical tips on how to make things better for our patients and the people we work with.

Bibliography

Berwick, D. (2013). *A Promise to Learn – A Commitment to Act: Improving the Safety of Patients in England.* London, UK: Department of Health and Social Care.

Committee on Quality of Health Care in America. (2001). *Crossing the Quality Chasm: A New Health System for the 21st Century.* Washington, DC: National Academy Press.

21

What could be better?

In this chapter, we will explore these questions:

- Do we know what high quality care looks like?
- How can we 'see ourselves as others see us'?
- Is it really possible to welcome complaints?

Identifying a quality issue

This section will focus on the first stage of any quality improvement (QI) process; how we decide what needs to be improved.

Generally, we're not very good at this. We think of new ideas or want to try something we have seen work in a practice or network down the road, but we don't spend time working out what problem it is *we* are trying to solve. As leaders of organisations we are often the people with the most enthusiasm for new ideas, and can be disappointed when others don't share our enthusiasm. This can sometimes be interpreted as a 'resistance to change'. This is sometimes true, but more often lack of enthusiasm for implementing a new idea can come from a lack of understanding of the purpose of the change. So, before introducing a new system (e.g., telephone triage, sending results by text, considering employing a practice pharmacist, etc. ...), be aware these are 'interventions'. We will only know if the interventions have succeeded if we have worked out what problem we are trying to solve in the first place.

Becoming better at noticing

The first step in deciding on an area for improvement relies on us noticing what is going on around us, and its impact. This is not as easy as it sounds. Every day we are overloaded with information to process and tasks to 'get done'. Noticing areas for improvement requires us to be better at seeing the detail in our everyday activities, and what goes on in our practice around us.

Noticing the detail in our working day is an undervalued task, and unless we make time for it, it usually doesn't happen. We are likely to be unable to do it effectively whilst we are also getting on with our day-to-day work. It turns out there is no such thing as the ability to multi-task. Multi-tasking involves engaging in two tasks simultaneously; in this case carrying out a work-related task at the same time as noticing the detail and spotting areas for improvement. The human brain can only effectively do one task at a time, unless one of the tasks is so well learnt to be automatic, like eating or walking. When we think we are multitasking, we are actually serial tasking. Rather than doing two things at once, we are switching from task to task in rapid succession. This has been shown to be much less efficient and effective that focussing on one task.

High workload, multiple interruptions and external distractions will all affect what we notice going on around us. We can also be internally distracted by our own thoughts, especially if we are suffering from stress or are dealing with negative emotions or adverse events.

The layout of our working environment and working patterns will also influence what we observe. The GPs and practice managers who rarely leave their consulting room or office will have fewer opportunities to spot processes that could be improved.

If we accept that noticing the details in our working day is a task in itself, it's clear we need to take some time out to do it, rather than assume it will happen whilst we are working on other things. It doesn't have to be time-consuming; sometimes just five minutes each day is enough. Remember it is just time out to 'notice', not to actually solve the issue. We don't need to make sense of the observations on our own; in fact, it's better if we don't. Just capture the thought and create an opportunity to discuss it with others later.

Tips for getting better at noticing

- Take active steps to avoid trying to 'multitask'
- Be aware when we are distracted by internal emotions or stresses and take time to look after ourselves
- Take time out each day to observe work being done by our team
- Ask questions to deeply understand the processes

Helping the team get better at noticing

It's fair to state that some people seem to be more observant than others and therefore, are more likely to notice things that could be better. Whether we observe something happening is one thing, whether we recognise the thing we observe could be having a negative impact, or could be improved, is another thing altogether.

How much people notice, and whether they decide the issue is important enough to highlight as an area for improvement can be influenced by what response they have had to similar activity in the past. The theory of operant conditioning suggests our behaviours are influenced by the outcome. So if the response to our action is positive, this reinforces the behaviour for the future. Positive reinforcement can be something as straightforward as praise or financial reward. However, seeing the impact of our suggestions on our organisation can act as powerful reinforcement. Highlighting an issue, that then leads to no further discussion or change will mean the person is less likely to notice things in the future.

There are a number of factors that influence how observant we are, whether we notice the possible impact of what we observe and then whether we decide to raise what we have noticed as a potential area for improvement.

Many general practice and primary care environments have had a stable staffing team for years, sometimes decades. Whilst there are advantages in stability and continuity, habits and ways of working can become ingrained and entrenched and people stop noticing waste or areas for improvement. Introducing new members of the team, or giving temporary members of the team, such as GP specialty trainees, medical students or student nurses permission to observe and comment on processes can be a valuable opportunity to view our practice through a 'fresh pair of eyes'.

Visiting different practices has taught us that there is a wide range of attitudes and behaviours amongst GPs, practice managers, and staff. These form part of the 'organisational culture' of the practice (see Chapter 1) and have generally built up over years. As a result, there are widely different thresholds for what is perceived to be 'good enough' and therefore, not spotted as an area for improvement. When a new person joins the team, they may spot areas for improvement, but unless they are invited to share their observations, they may be reticent to do so. After time they may acquire the habits of the rest of the team and the opportunity is missed.

> ## Tips for helping our team to notice areas for improvement
>
> - Positively reinforce the behaviour by taking notice of what team members observe
> - Don't be tempted to justify current practice or come to solutions too quickly, this may discourage future observations
> - Make the most of new or temporary team members as a 'fresh set of eyes' who can view a practice system or process problem that may have become a blind-spot to the rest of the team

Noticing an area for potential improvement is an important first step. It can be tempting to rush to a solution, and in certain, usually rare, circumstances the solution is obvious. Noticing, for example, that we are spending time constantly going upstairs to fetch something that is in regular use both upstairs and downstairs, like a laminator or shredder, can result in the conclusion that it would be worth buying another (provided the cost wasn't prohibitive). A simple solution to a simple problem. However, most things we spot will be more complex, multi-factorial issues that affect different team members in different ways. These issues need deeper levels of thinking before planning improvements; later in this section we will share tools and methods to do this. The important task at this stage is to capture what has been observed, prioritise its urgency depending on the harm of the current process and the potential benefit to patients and staff of sorting it.

Pause for thought – think about how you could capture this on a day-to-day basis in your practice?

A story about curiosity

We all know that curiosity is at the heart of all learning. Curious children learn quickly if provided with the right environment to do so. Quality improvement is a constant learning process and so curiosity is also at the heart of this.

We want to share a story, however true it is, that was heard in a talk about improvement. It's all about a man who gets a job for the civil service and starts to work at Whitehall. He is keen to maintain physical fitness so decides to cycle to work. On his first day, he arrives in the foyer with his cycle clips still on and carrying his helmet to be greeted by the doorman who calls him over to the desk and presents him with a signing in book. He says, 'I can see you have cycled to work Sir, so you need to sign in'. He diligently signs in and goes up to his office. The following day he arrived again and goes across to the desk to sign in but has noticed that other people arriving to work are and not being asked to sign the book. So he asks the doorman, 'I notice other people don't have to sign, why do I?' The doorman replies, 'Well, you are a cyclist sir, people who cycle to work sign in, sir'. When the man asks why, the doorman replies, 'Well, I'm not sure sir, but I shall find out for you'. The following day the man presents himself again at the desk to be met by the doorman who says, 'It turns out you don't have to sign in sir, you can go straight to the lift after all'. The doorman had discovered that during the war people who cycle to work were entitled extra rations at lunchtime, for which a register was needed, and so the habit continued for decades, unchallenged.

This is a lovely story, not only of how we can get stuck in our ways and do things long after the reason for them no longer exists. It can take somebody who is curious and with a fresh pair of eyes to spot a potential improvement.

What do others notice about us?

Working in a public service such as health care means that, as well as our own observations, our practice is observed by our patients, peers, regulators and external bodies who receive data about our performance. This feedback and data can 'hold a mirror' up to our processes and outcomes and give us clues on areas we might want to look at in more depth. Let's look at this in more detail.

Learning from patient complaints and feedback

Barlow and Moller's book on customer loyalty, *A Complaint Is a Gift* focussed on the value of negative feedback in helping us to fully understand our service and where there might be room for improvement. Working in a small to medium public sector organisation like a general practice it is very difficult for us to view complaints in this way for a variety of reasons:

- If the complaint is about the behaviour of an individual, the person involved can feel upset and fearful of blame, which can then generate self-doubt and adversely affect their performance or mental well-being.
- Complaints may affect reputation and have implications for performance reviews such as appraisal and revalidation.
- Staff are already working in challenging circumstances, and may feel unable to provide care to meet the expectations of patients and carers.

- The formal complaints procedure takes time out of an already busy working day for GPs and practice managers.
- Often complaints relate to the complex processes that operate across the health system and so feel to be out of the sole control of the practice.

Leaders have a role in helping to minimise the adverse impact of a complaint, and to identify aspects that could be used to generate positive improvement that would benefit all. We have a challenge here. As leaders we are also human, and complaints rarely generate positive emotions in any of us. Before we can help minimise the adverse psychological impact on the person named in the complaint, we need to first manage our own response, to try to stay as open-minded and rational as possible. Once we feel in control of our own responses, then it's time to gather information from those involved in the complaint, being aware their initial reactions are likely to be coloured by a whole range of emotions including anger and fear. Initial reactions fade, and sometimes just letting a bit of time pass can help everyone feel able to think more clearly and judge the issue as a useful learning event.

This will only work in practice if we have managed to create a learning culture, rather than a blame culture when things go wrong. The rush to blame may look decisive. It may seem like people are being held account-able for when things go wrong. In fact, the opposite can happen. Most events involve more than one person in the chain and usually involve pro-cess issues as well as people issues. By pinning the blame on individuals, we sometimes miss the bigger challenge of identifying the problems that often lurk in our complex systems.

It can be easy to overlook more informal comments and feedback from patients, both good and bad, which can help us identify areas for improve-ment. This could be a passing comment made by a patient at the front desk or in the consultation room or the more formalised 'friends and family test' that operates through many health services. This involves patients/carers being asked to answer the question, 'How likely are you to recommend our service to friends and family if they needed similar care or treatment?', followed by the opportunity to free text a reason for the chosen ranking. There can be so much variation in response rate from one month to the next it is difficult to make sense of the quantitative data; the free text com-ments, however, are more likely to provide a source of opportunities for you to see your practice through the eyes of those who use it.

We are now in an age of constant requests for feedback and everyone has an opportunity to be a critic or reviewer. After every online purchase we are asked to review the product that we have bought. Our patients (and others) are increasingly likely to post their thoughts about our practices publicly rather than sharing this privately with us. Some feedback may be posted anonymously, so there is always a possibility a complainant may not have had any real interaction with our practice. The practice is not always aware that a comment has been posted, and there is often no mechanism for responding. This can be frustrating and distressing for practices if the comment is negative, and this can make it more difficult to view the feedback as a potentially useful observation that can identify an area for improvement. Sometimes we need to give ourselves permission to ignore this type of feedback, especially if the main intention appears to be to cause offense. Our role as leaders in this situation is to spot trends or patterns. Sometimes it is easy to forget the hundreds of patient interactions that occur smoothly every week and to focus too much on a single vexatious social media comment.

Learning from benchmarking

Comparing our performance with others can help us pick up on areas for improvement. Various organisations collect data about our practices and our performance, which we can use for benchmarking to decide if we have an area that might need some work. Some of this data may be easily accessible from public websites, and the range of available data will vary depending on where you work.

Examples of areas of our practice performance that can be compared with others include:

- Prescribing data (e.g., the number of antibiotics prescribed per 1000 patients)
- Childhood immunisation rates
- Cancer screening data (the uptake on cervical, breast, and bowel cancer)
- Patient satisfaction
- Cancer diagnosis data, including the number of cancers that have been diagnosed using the recommended fast-track referral procedure
- Admission rates for a variety of specified conditions
- Referral rates to secondary care
- Achievement of the recommended processes of care and treatment targets for our patients with diabetes
- Rates of missed appointments

All benchmarking data needs to be viewed in context, as there may be some justifiable reason why our performance varies from our peer practices. Benchmarking data is sometimes used by external bodies for quality assurance purposes (rather than for improvement) and so we find ourselves in a position of needing to explain variation to our commissioners, health boards or regulators who may not be aware of our practice context. However, it is easy to fall into the habit of justifying variation in order to avoid criticism, or because we have a blind spot. As improvement is a process we need to own, we can challenge our usual habits of justification and compare ourselves with practices we know to have a similar demographic and morbidity.

Benchmarking data can be presented in a variety of ways, depending on the level of statistical analysis. The most straightforward presentation is a column graph, usually arranged from the most highly performing practice on one side, to the least well-performing practice on the other. Sometimes these graphs will also include the locality (in this case CCG) or national average performance.

Example of benchmarking data

Percentage of patients saying it is 'easy' to get through to someone on the phone.

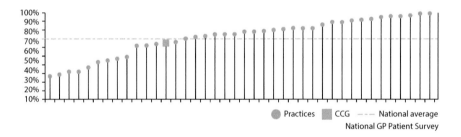

Practices   CCG   – – – National average
National GP Patient Survey

Displaying performance data in this way has the advantage of simplicity but fails to reflect the importance of sample size when deciding if the variation in the data is a true reflection of the variation in performance. If we are genuinely interested in knowing if our telephone access needs to improve, we might use this data as a starting point but then seek out other sources of information such as patient informal feedback or conduct our own survey.

It is important to be aware of the limitations of this type of data. Externally sourced data is often 12 to 18 months old by the time it reaches the public domain, so may not reflect any recent changes or improvements we have made.

Another criticism of using 'benchmarking' to decide if improvements are needed is that it encourages mediocrity: being in the middle range is acceptable. If we just use benchmarking to find areas for improvement, we lose the opportunity to explore just how good our performance could be if we tried something new.

Learning from peers and networks

Across the NHS in the United Kingdom there is an increasing emphasis on practices working together in networks (the name of these groups varies across the four nations of the United Kingdom) to provide care for the patients of a defined geographical population. Although the purpose of a network is wide-ranging, it provides opportunities for GPs and practice managers to learn from each other. Practices develop their own processes and habits over decades, and as a result it is hard to see that there is ever an alternative way of working. When leading group discussions with leaders from different practices we often witness 'light-bulb' moments, when one PM or GP hears about a way of working that they had never thought of, that improves patient experience and reduces workload.

Although there are opportunities from finding out about how others run their processes, there are also potential pitfalls. Although it can be tempting to take the great idea we have just heard about straight back to our practices and introduce it, good quality improvement (QI) is rarely just about the good idea and needs us to fully understand our own practice context and understand the problem we are trying to solve. (See case study later in this chapter.) Effective QI usually needs the local team to 'own their own solution', even if the initial trigger for the change has come from seeing how things are done elsewhere. However, if we hear about a good idea from a peer, we can put the time aside to visit the practice and see the idea in action in their context, and ask deeper questions, ideally with other key leaders with whom we work.

Earlier in this chapter, we discussed the importance of noticing, and how this can sometimes be more effective when new people join the team. Being part of a local network of practices gives opportunities for us to invite in a 'fresh pair of eyes', to see our service and ask questions and thereby help us to understand it better. If a GP or practice manager from another practice in our network spent a day with us, what would they see? Give them permission to give honest feedback.

Over the stile

We get so embedded in our own organisational cultures; it can be very hard, unless something major occurs, for us to be able to identify what could be better. Then, once we develop better awareness, we can then feel overwhelmed by the sheer number of things we want to change. Neither state is ideal. In the next chapter, we explore how to get to the bottom of why things are as they are, so that we don't attempt to fix the wrong things and also how to prioritise, in a world where nothing will ever be perfect.

Bibliography

Barlow, J. & Moller, C. (2008). *A Complaint Is a Gift: Recovering Customer Loyalty When Things Go Wrong* (2nd ed.). Berrett-Koehler Publishers.

NHS England. *National GP Patient Survey.* https://www.gp-patient.co.uk/.

22

Understand the problem

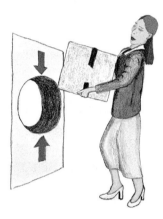

Understanding the problem

In the previous chapter, we looked at how we might notice when things aren't quite right about the quality of our service or the care we are providing.

If we decide there may be room for improvement, there can be a number of different responses. We might:

- Decide the issue is not solvable, or blame an external agent. This can happen if it has been identified by externally gathered data, especially if we decide the data is flawed,
- Attempt to immediately fix the issue ourselves,
- Delegate the fix to someone else in the practice, who may or may not have the skills to fix it,
- Fear the problem seems too big to change and allow inertia to set in,
- Decide the problem is not within our power to improve and do nothing.

An alternative approach is to realise we have only identified the issue, and there is more we need to do to fully understand it, in order to know the best way forward.

Our role as leaders is to recognise the value in gaining a deeper and broader understanding of the problem areas and be able to communicate this to others. We need to hold the conversation open for long enough to give others a chance to participate in gaining this understanding as this will be the foundations of engaging others in the solution.

Case study – Improving access to same day care

Practice Y had struggled with the demand for same day GP appointments for years. In an attempt to solve this, five years previously, they had implemented a daily morning walk-in surgery. Although this seemed to help at first, they were now working through lunch and the waiting room was constantly full of patients who had often been waiting for 2–3 hours. The GPs were hungry and stressed.

At a locality meeting on of the partners, Dr J, heard about the 'telephone first' system that a neighbouring practice had implemented. Every person who requested an appointment with a GP was booked a phone consultation first. The practice had been pleased with the results and found that fewer people needed to be seen face-to-face and patients received more prompt care, sometimes being signposted to a more appropriate service.

(Continued)

After weeks of trying to implement a similar system back at Practice Y, the practice was in chaos. The patients were much less happy with the new system. Many patients had English as their second language and found it difficult to explain their symptoms over the phone. There weren't enough phone lines to cope with all the calls, so the lines were constantly engaged. The GPs weren't used to telephone consulting and found it more stressful than the old system. Patients were dealt with more quickly than in the old system, but patient satisfaction fell.

In the case study, it's worth reflecting on what problem it was they were trying to solve by implementing the telephone first solution. It could have been:

- GPs getting a lunch break
- GP stress levels
- Time patients spend in the waiting room
- Patients getting the right care at the right time
- Patient satisfaction with waiting time

If the QI process had started by exploring and deciding exactly which problem or problems they were trying to fix, there was significantly more chance they would have developed a solution to better fit the problem. There is always more than one solution, and the best solution will be the one we, our teams and our patients have designed and tested.

Participative QI tools can help teams gain a better understanding of why practice performance or outcomes may not be what we aspire to. They can help us to decide what changes we might want to try out when we start the process of improvement. Additionally, tools can depersonalise, make the influence on decision-making more objective and encourage leaders to ask the questions, rather than give answers. Our role is to select tools appropriately and facilitate them with care, so that our teams feel fully involved in the process. Using formal QI 'diagnosis' tools takes time, so we need to choose wisely.

The table below lists eight tools that have been used in general practice to 'diagnose' improvement needs prior to embarking on a QI project. We rarely need to use all of them; different tools are useful for different purposes and they can all be adapted if needed.

TOOL FOR 'DIAGNOSIS'	BEST USED TO EXPLORE	PURPOSE
Significant Event Audit	A single issue	To deepen the understanding of why something happened
5 Whys	A single issue that keeps occurring	To deepen the understanding of why something happens repeatedly
Fishbone Diagram	A single issue that is impacted by many factors	To deepen and broaden the understanding when an issue is multi-factoral
Process Mapping	A process that has multiple steps, and involving multiple people that all work together to achieve the right outcome	To achieve a shared understanding of the problem areas and wasted steps
Appreciative Inquiry	Could be used for anything from a single issue, to the whole practice or network	To focus our attention on what we do well; to build on areas of strength
Forcefield Analysis	A single issue	To look at the pros or cons of making a change, or introducing a new service
SWOT Analysis	A single issue	To broaden our view of a potential change for the practice before a decision is made
PESTLE Analysis	To take a wider view	To spot opportunities for positive change and plan for potential threats to our service

Significant Event Audit (SEA)/learning from incidents

SEA is used to explore areas for potential improvement in more depth. The traditional model for conducting an SEA has seven stages:

1 Identifying and prioritising
2 Information gathering
3 Facilitated team-based meeting
4 Analysis of the event (What happened? Why did it happen? What has been learned? What changes are needed?)
5 Agree, implement and monitor change
6 Write up the event/learning
7 Share the learning more widely if appropriate

The GPs and their teams have been encouraged to identifying incidents in practice and consider conducting SEAs. The examples could include:

CLINICAL INCIDENT	PRESCRIBING INCIDENT	ADMINISTRATIVE INCIDENT	UNPLANNED WORK OR REWORK
New diagnoses of cancer	Wrong drug prescribed	Clinic letter misfiled	Patient arrived but not checked in
Unexpected death	Wrong drug dose	Wrong result given over the phone	Clinician phoned in sick
Positive cervical smear	Inadequate drug monitoring	Important message not acted on	Locum didn't turn up
Positive mammography	Drug monitoring test not acted on	Result filed without being acted on	Unannounced extra patient left in waiting room
Intentional overdose/ self-harm	Drug interaction not noticed	Urgent referral not done	Patient aggressive at the front desk
Asthma admission to hospital	Misinterpretation of a handwritten prescription request	Appointment letter sent to wrong address	
Misinterpretation of a result	Acute drug reissued as repeat	Investigation request not sent	
Unplanned pregnancy	Poor INR control	Referral letter not sent	
Patient collapsed after procedure	Drug interaction not noticed	Home visit forgotten	
No trainer to cover GP Specialist trainee	Medication not reconciled following admission	Home visit to the wrong address	
Failure to follow up abnormal result		Text sent to wrong mobile number	

There is a good evidence to suggest that many SEAs are not conducted well by practice teams for a range of reasons. Being involved in a significant event can feel similar to receiving a complaint. The emotional response can get in the way of the individuals being able to see beyond their own failure so they struggle to be objective about the factors that led to the event. It can contribute to feelings of stress, anxiety and guilt impacting on mental well-being.

Although organisations effective at continuous learning and improvement aim to have a 'no blame' culture, it is relatively unusual to find this in practice. There is still widespread fear of punishment or professional embarrassment, which has an impact on which events are chosen for analysis, limiting the usefulness of the process. During the analysis there is often too much focus on the actions of individuals who are perceived to have made an error. The individuals themselves tend to view the 'causes' of incidents as being mainly attributable to their own actions or inactions with is largely contrary to human error theory. SEA research shows there are often wider system 'contributory factors' involved.

Some of the common actions that result following a SEA are:

- Write a protocol
- More staff training
- Staff to read the practice protocol
- Staff to follow protocol more consistently

These actions fail to recognise the complexities that lie behind human error. Paul Bowie and colleagues, in their work on Enhanced SEA in Scotland, considered incidents occurring due to an interaction between:

- *People factors,* including being over-tired, distracted, interrupted, and relying too heavily on limited human memory and attention span.
- *Activity factors,* including recent alterations to process, such as new immunisation schedules, too many steps in a process, lots of repetition of a task with some variation, drugs with very similar names, immunisations in similar-looking boxes.
- *Environment factors,* including cluttered desks, poorly design cupboard/fridge storage, IT systems lacking built in safety features, such as prescribing alerts.

Breaking down the 'Why did it happen?' stage of the SEA can help the team be more objective and constructive when understanding causes, and therefore be able to develop more useful system-level changes that don't simply rely on everyone getting better at remembering, or concentrating more, or becoming better at following protocol.

More training or a brilliant protocol does not necessary result in safe error-free practice. Historically, there has been an over-reliance on protocol as a way of describing work as it 'should' be carried out. People don't always do the 'right thing', and sometimes with good reason. The reality is that working in healthcare is often muddled and unpredictable with multiple non-linear relationships and interactions between people that are taking place all of the time. To really understand this, we need to pay attention to what is actually happening in practice as a result of people working with each other, rather than being enslaved to beliefs about what we think ought to happen according to our protocols.

We wouldn't suggest leaders reject SEA altogether as a tool for improving care, just that they understand its limitations and try out alternative, more agile methods for understanding problem areas.

We have tended to focus on problems in isolation, one harm at a time, and our efforts have been simplistic and myopic. If we are to save more lives and significantly reduce patient harm, we need to adopt a holistic, systematic approach that extends across cultural, technological and procedural boundaries – one that is based on the evidence of what works.

Professor the Lord Ara Darzi

SEA case study

Mrs B had recently attended her rheumatology appointment and brought in a handwritten request from her consultant for her GP to prescribe Sulfasalazine 500 mg. The receptionist explained the practice policy that non-urgent prescriptions would be available after three working days. The patient was well-known to the practice and was struggling with her arthritis. She explained that the following morning she was going on a trip to France for four weeks to visit her sister and asked if the prescription could possibly be made available later the same day. The receptionist said she would see if it could be done as urgent.

She took the request in to Dr S, who was on call, and explained the situation. Dr S was about 1 hour behind with her on-call duties and had just received a request for three home visits at the local care home. She could see the handwriting on the request was poor but was fairly sure it read Sulfadiazine 500 mg. She prescribed this (an incorrect drug) and the prescription was sent electronically to the pharmacy. Various alerts came up about this being an antibiotic, but Dr S

(*Continued*)

dismissed them, as alerts always 'pop up' whenever she prescribed rheumatology drugs, and very few of the alerts are meaningful.

The pharmacist thought this was an unusual prescription, and as it was for an antibiotic used infrequently, they were going to need to order it from their suppliers, and it wouldn't be arriving until later in the day. They decided to query it with Dr S, but when they tried to phone the practice the phone line was constantly engaged. Mrs B was understandably anxious to get her medication before her trip to France and so assured the pharmacist that she was sure it *was* the right drug.

The wrong drug was dispensed.

Outcome of poorly led SEA meeting

It is easy to see how a poorly run SEA meeting can result in a serious of 'shoulds' or 'should nevers':

- Consultants **should** print all their medication requests clearly
- The practice **should** have a new policy of only issuing non-urgent prescriptions in response to a typed request
- Receptionists **should never** promise to rush prescriptions through the system, they **should always** follow protocol
- GPs **should never** ignore prescribing safety alerts
- Pharmacists **should** always check out concerns with the prescriber before dispensing

This is a typical example of the 'must try harder' outcome that can come out of many SEA meetings. It leaves the receptionist, GP, and pharmacist feeling blamed and responsible for factors embedded within a system. For leaders, this is a cop-out. It means that we don't have to look more deeply at our systems and ask questions that could result in improvements which could benefit all.

In this example, all the receptionists' job was to respond kindly to a patient's needs. The GP was trying to multi-task to meet all the demands on her at that time, and had become blind to prescribing alerts because the system generated so many it was hard to see the wood for the trees. The pharmacist's actions were influenced by his own workload and the difficulties in accessing the practice by phone.

As health care is a people business, there will always be people with poor handwriting, and people whose outpatient appointments fall just before their holidays. There's probably not much we can do about this, and certainly it's not something a policy or protocol will help to solve. Instead, this event raises questions about the duties of the on-call doctor, the threshold for prescribing safety alerts, the practice telephone system and the ways in which the pharmacists can contact the practice at short notice.

Tips for leading 'learning from incidents'

- Be sensitive to the feelings of those involved in the incident. Help everyone to understand the purpose of a SEA is to look at the bigger picture, not individual failings
- Use events as an opportunity to build a culture of continuous learning, openness, candour and belonging
- Be prepared to share your own vulnerability
- Prioritise incidents for full analysis, but try out other methods of learning
- If you find 'must try harder' is the endpoint of your SEAs, then find ways of helping your team think more creatively about solutions.

5 Whys

The *5 Whys* technique was originally developed by Sakichi Toyoda and was used by the Toyota Motor Corporation during the evolution of its manufacturing methods. The simple act of asking 'why' in a structured participative way can uncover important factors related to human behaviour and our working environment that contribute to either poor performance or inefficient processes and systems. The method involves repeatedly asking the question 'Why' (five is often a useful target to aim for); each answer will lead us to another question until we get to the root cause of the problem. Although this technique is called '5 Whys', you may find that you will need to ask the question fewer or more times than five before you find the issue related to a problem.

The '5 Whys' approach is particularly useful when a single issue keeps recurring. Examples include:

- Running out of a consumable, for example, bed roll or printer ink
- Prescriptions being sent to the wrong pharmacy
- Letters being scanned onto the wrong electronic medical record
- Medication reviews not being updated once blood results are back
- Sick notes ('Fit notes') not being ready when patients come to collect them

5 Whys example

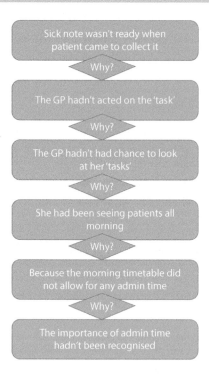

Sick note wasn't ready when patient came to collect it

Why?

The GP hadn't acted on the 'task'

Why?

The GP hadn't had chance to look at her 'tasks'

Why?

She had been seeing patients all morning

Why?

Because the morning timetable did not allow for any admin time

Why?

The importance of admin time hadn't been recognised

The technique not only helps identify the root cause of a problem but also the relationship between different root causes of a problem. It is a particularly useful technique when problems involve human factors or interactions and when there are simple, linear reasons behind a problem. It is less helpful in exploring complex, multi-factoral problems. In this situation, the '5 Whys' approach can be expanded and structured in the form of a fishbone diagram.

Fishbone diagram

Fishbone diagrams are also known as Ishikawa or 'cause and effect' diagrams. They work most effectively when constructed by several members of a team who want to explore a problem area. The exercise helps generate a shared understanding of the problem, when multiple factors may be contributing. It helps to ensure important potential factors are not ignored and at the same time it sorts ideas into useful categories. It can be a useful alternative to using a SEA approach, as it can feel less 'personal'.

Examples of problems that can be explored by constructing a fishbone diagram include:

- Lost prescriptions
- Overdue review dates
- Surgeries over-running
- Results not actioned
- Worsening cervical smear performance

How to create a fishbone diagram:

1   Identify the problem, which becomes the head of the fish.
2   Ask the group to think of the main categories of causes of the problem. In this example shown these are patient, doctor, nurse/HCA, organisation and resources, although you may think of others. These form the spines of the fish.
3   Discuss each major category, adding the ideas generated as sub-branches. Each sub-branch may be further broken down into its contributing factors.
4   For every spine and sub-branch identified, ask yourself 'Why does this happen?' and consider the question from different perspectives – such as patient, administrator, nurse, doctor and commissioner. This will produce the layers of causes that will help you to fully understand the root of the problem and its dependencies.
5   Use your completed diagram to help you to generate ideas for improvement.

Fishbone diagram example: Why do we have a high number of patients with poor blood pressure control?

Step 1:

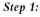

Step 2:

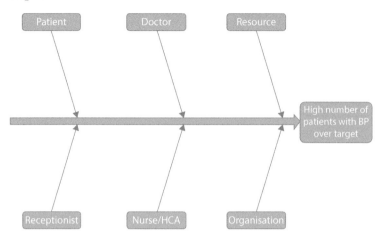

Step 3:

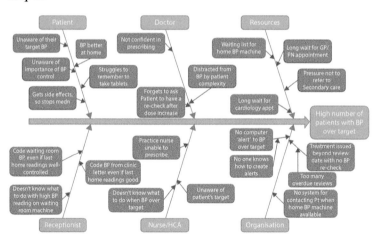

Process mapping

The delivery of health care to our patients is complex and could be described as a web of different internal and external processes that interface with each other, often seemingly with little co-ordination. In general practice, we work with a wide range of processes including:

- Repeat prescribing
- Patients accessing appointments

- Referrals
- Managing incoming mail
- Long-term condition reviews
- New patient registrations
- Managing investigation results

Any problem within these processes can affect the quality of care we offer and the outcomes for our patients and can generate waste and rework for our practice teams. It's not always easy to see where the real problem lies within a process without an understanding of the process from start to finish, and from the perspective of everyone involved in the process, including our patients and carers. Process mapping is a group exercise that results in the creation of a visual map of the process, with the problem areas being identified.

How to create a process map

The process mapping exercise needs to be actively facilitated, but special expertise isn't needed, just the ability to encourage people to participate. It's helpful if the facilitator only adds their own contribution once they have heard from others. It often works well if the facilitator doesn't have a good understanding of the process to be mapped. Invite anyone involved in the process to participate in the mapping exercise, including patients who interact with the process. Post-it notes of at least two colours and pens will be needed.
   During the session:

- *Step 1:* The facilitator explains process mapping to the participants, making it clear that each step needs to be broken down. The more detailed the better because this will identify waste.
- *Step 2:* Define the start and end point of the process. For managing results, you could start with identifying a patient needs an investigation and end with the patient being aware of the result and what it means.
- *Step 3:* If one step can be done in several ways, this is added vertically, for example, in the repeat prescribing process the patient may request a script in different ways.
- *Step 4:* Once the map is created, the facilitator asks the group where the problems arise, or steps that seem to have no purpose. The participants then note the problems on a different coloured Post-it note and attach these at the appropriate point on the map.

- **Step 5:** Participants are then asked to identify solutions. These are noted on another different coloured Post-it note. They are stuck over the problems that were identified.
- **Step 6:** This process will then have identified areas for improvement and generated new ideas to try out.
- **Step 7:** A further process map is then created by the group to illustrate the agreed new process.

By the end, you will have created a visual display of an improvement to an existing process. The exercise often highlights the more steps there are a process, the more likely it is there is inefficiency. It is a good idea to leave the map on display for a few weeks so that any issues that arise during implementation can be more easily discussed.

Process mapping helps a team gain a shared understanding and this has a positive impact on how well people engage with the improvement plan. If we try to improve processes without this understanding, we can suggest changes that may seem sensible from our perspective but fail to recognise the impact of our suggestion on other aspects of the process. Just creating the map helps to change attitudes and the process mapping exercise therefore serves two purposes, both helping us to understand the problem areas and engaging the team in the improvement process which follows.

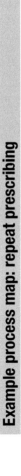

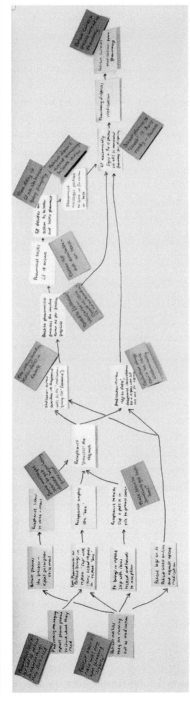

Example process map: repeat prescribing

Photo Credit: Adam Bircher

Appreciative inquiry

When leading change in an organisation, a positive, optimistic outlook can help to encourage and engage others to take part. However, this chapter so far has been focussed on how we notice and explore things that may be going wrong; a deficit-based approach. Getting better at noticing problem areas can have a negative impact on the mood of a team, leading to a sense of doom and gloom or frustration that things never seem to get any better. The more we notice and focus on what has gone wrong, the more the difficulty become all that we see.

In the 1980s, a group of business consultants working in the United States (Ohio) with a hotel in difficulties recognised that the deficit-based approach was resulting in an overwhelming sense of hopelessness amongst the hotel leaders and staff. They decided to try out a new approach and then formalised this into a process now known as appreciative inquiry (AI).

> AI involves, at its root, the art and practice of crafting questions that support a system's capacity to apprehend, anticipate, and heighten positive potential. The AI is a quest to discover the 'positive core' of a system – the past, present, and future capacities to cooperate for the common good.
>
> **Barrett, Fry and Wittock, 2005**

Although we include AI in this section on 'understanding the problem', using the method we reach a better understanding of our practice, but by taking a different and entirely positive approach. It is a complementary way of understanding the factors relevant to the better outcomes we seek and can be particularly helpful when we find ourselves facing multiple challenges and at times of low morale.

The AI is not about solving problems; it is about inquiring into what works well in order to build on the strengths of the people and the organisation.

DEFICIT STATEMENTS/INQUIRY	APPRECIATIVE INQUIRY
What's the main problem?	Which part of this process works really well?
Why is this not working?	What does our 'best day' look like?
What are the barriers?	What made it go well on that occasion?
That won't work because …	How can we develop more of this?
We should have done that differently.	The right way to do this is …
We've tried that before.	It could work even better if we …

(Adapted from Wiggins, L. and Hunter, H., *Relational Change: The Art and Practice of Changing Organizations*, Bloomsbury Business, 2016.)

Practical AI tips

- When running a meeting to plan implementing change, start by creating a timeline of the practice including significant achievements and changes you have successfully navigated in the past
- Try to capture a positive story of patient care well-delivered to share at every team meeting
- Develop new appreciative inquiry questions and remember to use them often
- Make sure the whole team is aware when a positive comment about the practice is received or posted on-line

The AI is not about trying to pretend problems don't occur, or papering over the cracks. Nor is it about wishful thinking, as it is based on real examples of positive events in the past or the present and allows the energy that emerges from focussing on the positive to be transferred to dreaming and designing an even better future.

Forcefield analysis

Even if we are convinced that implementing a change at the practice is a good idea, others may not, and they may have some reasonable concerns that need to be heard before any decision is made. A forcefield analysis is a tool to help us and the team decide whether to implement a change or not. It helps us as leaders to suspend judgement, giving ourselves long enough to be open-minded.

It often doesn't take long to carry out a forcefield analysis, and generally people are familiar with the concept of putting together a list of pros and cons. This tool merely formalises this process, adding some numerical values to the pros and cons in an attempt to achieve consensus about whether to go ahead or not.

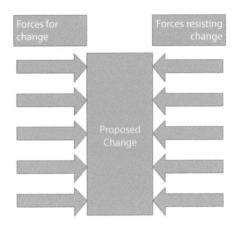

Step by step: how to lead a forcefield analysis

Step 1: Gather together as many people as you can who will be impacted by the change, including those implementing it.

Step 2: Ask the group to think of as many 'pros' and 'cons' as they can. They may want to write each one on a separate Post-it note, as not everyone feels comfortable saying their opinions out loud. The 'pros' are the forces for change, the 'cons' and the forces resisting the change.

Step 3: If there are strong feelings in the room, then take care to ensure you have spent enough time gathering all the 'pros' and 'cons'. If necessary, leave the lists up on a flip chart in a prominent place in the practice so that people can add to the list as they think of more factors.

Step 4: If there appear to be duplicates, then agree this with the group and just display one version.

Step 5: Arrange the forces for the change and the forces resisting the change on either side of the display board or flip chart.

Step 6: Agree a numerical value to each of the forces according to how much influence each has on the change being considered.

Step 7: Add up the total score for the forces on each side.

Step 8: Analyse.

Once you've done your force field analysis, you can use it to either decide whether or not to move forward with the change or to think about which supportive forces you can strengthen and which opposing or resisting forces you can weaken in order to make the change more successful.

Example of a forcefield analysis in action

A practice had become involved in a local initiative to encourage their patient group to develop activities to address some of the social determinants of poor health. They had welcomed the opportunity and started some initiatives aimed at older people who were socially isolated, and for those with low levels of physical activity. Both schemes were developing well and they now wanted to develop something for the young people in the area who were experiencing poor mental health. Their idea was to run an evening, once a week, for board games, for young people aged from 14 to 25.

When the idea was presented to the practice, the staff were very concerned about the impact of this on the practice and could think of many barriers. They carried out a forcefield analysis as shown in the illustration.

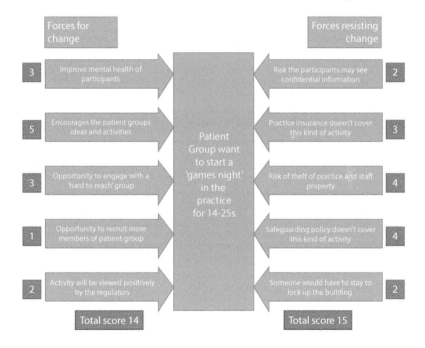

When they saw the scores, they realised the pros and cons were fairly well-balanced. They also recognised they could mitigate against some of the risks they identified. One of the members of the patient group was happy to look at the safeguarding policy to see what changes would be needed.

It wouldn't be appropriate to spend time on a forcefield analysis if we are aware that there is an absolute hurdle that must be overcome before a project can go ahead, for example, some aspects of the law that needed to be complied with. However, once we know that absolute barriers can be overcome, the analysis can prove useful to in disclosing other factors.

SWOT analysis

At times a forcefield analysis is too simple a tool to explore the possible impact of an external factor on our practice, and to look for opportunities. A SWOT analysis might be just what we are looking for. It is a tool designed to be used with a group of people, so that the practice can understand what it is good at, be more aware of weaknesses, be ready to exploit opportunities and mitigate against threats to our future. Here, SWOT stands for Strengths, Weaknesses, Opportunities, and Threats.

A SWOT analysis can help us to answer more complex questions such as:

- Should we become a training practice?
- Should we merge with the practice next door?
- Should we offer to be the lead practice in our network?

Step by step: how to lead a SWOT analysis

Step 1: Gather together people who will be impacted by the change.

Step 2: Explain the change that is being discussed; encourage questions and allow for a general discussion before starting the SWOT analysis. People will find it easier to participate if they have heard about some of the issues in more detail. This may have already been addressed if your SWOT analysis has followed on from a forcefield analysis.

Step 3: Explain the exercise and give some examples of what issue might fall into each category. Strengths and weaknesses are generally factors related to the practice and practice team, and opportunities and threats generally factors external to the practice. See the diagram.

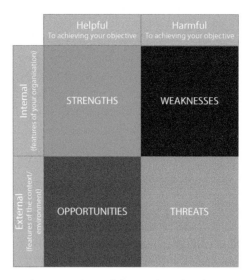

Step 4: Draw a large version of the grid in the diagram on a flip chart or a white board.

Step 5: Participants are given Post-it notes and are asked to write one item in each category.

Step 6: Ask for their Post-it notes, category by category, read them out, and stick them in the appropriate section on the grid. If there appear to be duplicates, agree this with the group and just include one of the Post-its.

Step 7: Ask the group to look at the grid particularly thinking of any areas that have not been covered by the existing Post-its and to write more Post-its to fill the gaps. One idea per Post-it note.

Step 8: Repeat Step 6, ensuring that by the end of the exercise all participants have shared their thoughts.

Step 9: Reflection of the exercise. Ask the group the following questions:

- *What do you notice on the grid?* Try to encourage the participants to not jump to conclusions at this point and just objectively state what they notice.

- *How do you feel when you see what we have created?* Getting in touch with how we feel about something can be an important part of decision making. Does the grid make them feel excited? Or fearful? Linking in with our emotional responses can be helpful in deepening reflection and can lead to better decision making.

- *How do you make sense of this?* Changing anything requires energy. Making sense of our emotional responses can help us to identify if we have the energy to carry through the change, and which may be the most significant barriers.

- *How does this help us decide what to do next?*
- *What could we do next?* Using the word 'could' means we don't close down the decision-making process too soon. There is still time for options to be explored, especially if we don't yet know if the 'threats' are real, or if the 'weaknesses' can be addressed.

Example of SWOT analysis

You would like to set up a coil clinic at your practice. You bring this up at a practice meeting and it triggers a heated debate with conflicting opinions about the benefits.

Dr Anna is keen as she has recently learned how to fit coils and knows she needs to fit at least 12 every year to maintain her competence and accreditation.

Dr Brian used to fit coils but gave up having had some bad experiences with complications, which knocked his confidence and made him feel vulnerable to litigation. He doesn't want to put anyone else in this position.

Joanne is the reception manager, and has noticed patients are very disappointed when they find out they need to travel five miles and wait three months for a coil-fitting at the local sexual health service.

Sarah is the practice business manager and priced up the cost of the equipment and staff time for a coil-fitting and noticed there was only a small margin of profit on each fitting, which would soon disappear if the price of the equipment or staff cost were to rise. She also manages the allocation of rooms, and this job is becoming harder since the practice employed a pharmacist and is supervising more medical students.

Joan is the practice manager. She is a good friend of the practice manager at a neighbouring practice, and aware they have a falling list size and are concerned about their long-term future. However, she is also aware that, when the practice is inspected, they will be assessed on how well they are meeting the needs of a range of patients, including those who need long-acting contraception.

Sue is the practice information manager, responsible for making claims for services. Every month she has to making several claims, all using different forms and processes. She has heard from a colleague that the coil claims are complex and she may have to chase up the reimbursement from the contractors frequently.

It is clear these is no consensus so you decide if it would be helpful to use a SWOT analysis to explore all the factors people are bringing up during the discussion:

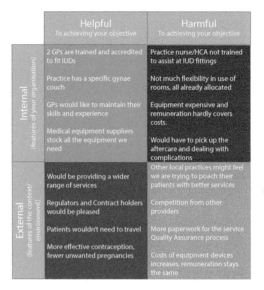

	Helpful To achieving your objective	Harmful To achieving your objective
Internal (features of your organisation)	2 GPs are trained and accredited to fit IUDs	Practice nurse/HCA not trained to assist at IUD fittings
	Practice has a specific gynae couch	Not much flexibility in use of rooms, all already allocated
	GPs would like to maintain their skills and experience	Equipment expensive and remuneration hardly covers costs.
	Medical equipment suppliers stock all the equipment we need	Would have to pick up the aftercare and dealing with complications
External (features of the context/environment)	Would be providing a wider range of services	Other local practices might feel we are trying to poach their patients with better services
	Regulators and Contract holders would be pleased	Competition from other providers
	Patients wouldn't need to travel	More paperwork for the service Quality Assurance process
	More effective contraception, fewer unwanted pregnancies	Costs of equipment devices increases, remuneration stays the same

The exercise went well and everyone felt heard. During the reflective conversation at the end (Step 9) it was clear there wasn't enough energy amongst your team to drive it forward. You felt less disappointed about this than you had expected once you heard the views of others.

However, when your team were asked 'What could we do next?', it was clear the 'strengths' and 'opportunities' had also been heard by all. The team decided to get together with the neighbouring practices to design a shared service. This would enable the GPs to maintain their skills, and provide a local service for the population, whilst sharing the bureaucracy and the risk.

PESTLE analysis

This tool was developed for businesses to enable them to take a 'bird's-eye' look at their organisation from a variety of different perspectives. PESTLE is an acronym, every letter standing for a different 'lens' through which to examine the organisation. It helps us to look at the bigger picture, consider working across boundaries and developing opportunities that help us to evolve beyond what's staring us in the face. It can be particularly useful to use this approach when the practice (or 'at-scale' organisation such as a network, cluster, neighbourhood or federation) is considering a major change in direction, or has spotted a big challenge on the horizon. The framework helps us to see the different forces that may be affecting our practice performance or the options open to us.

It is change, continuing change, inevitable change that is the dominant factor in society today. No sensible decision can be made any longer without taking into account not only the world as it is, but the world as it will be.

Isaac Asimov

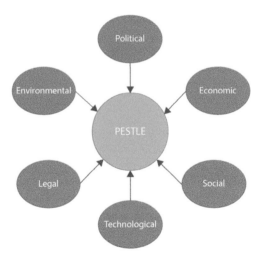

Examples of PESTLE factors affecting general practice

POLITICAL	ECONOMIC	SOCIAL	TECHNOLOGICAL	LEGAL	ENVIRONMENTAL
NHS policy	Inflation	Media campaigns	Electronic medical record	Contracting models	Air quality
NHS long-term plan	Cost of living	Public opinion	Patient access	External regulators	Increase in local house-building
Immigration policy affecting workforce	Investment in General Practice	Social attitudes	Patients informed by on-line searches	GP revalidation	Transport links
Degree of health and social care integration	Pension changes	Popularity of working in healthcare	Innovations to make work easier	Privacy legislation	Availability of green space
Elections and changes in government	Change to National Insurance	Community assets	Move to electronic referrals	Equalities Act	Availability of health and leisure facilities
GP contract changes		Ageing population			Closure of nearby practice

A PESTLE analysis is most useful if it is revisited often in order for the practice to scan the horizon for potential challenges so we can make preparations. It is so easy to spend all of our time focussing on the day-to-day running of our practices; the PESTLE framework encourages us to think outwardly. In reality, though, it is quite a time-consuming exercise and likely to be most useful when we are facing big challenges that may warrant major change in the structure of the organisations we lead. A PESTLE analysis can be a useful basis for the creation of a practice business plan.

Step by step PESTLE analysis

Step 1: Create your own list of factors within each category. The table is for ideas only; you are likely to think of others.

Step 2: Consider which are currently having or are likely to have the greatest impact on your practice.

Step 3: Consider how the factor is likely to create an impact, and whether this would be positive or negative, and how great the impact could be.

Step 4: Consider the timescale for the impact.

Step 5: Decide if any action is needed to either encourage positive change, or mitigate the risk of a negative impact.

The choices we make

This section has been quite detailed on tools, and seemingly less about our role as leaders. However, the part we play is so important. Although it is useful to know about the tools, their effectiveness is dependent on choosing well and using well. Using these tools effectively is more akin to learning to dance, than learning to follow a recipe and improves with practice. It pulls in our best listening and communication skills, our ability to welcome and respect a diversity of views and to hold an open mind, allowing our own ideas to be challenged and changed by the exercise.

Improvement doesn't just involve making choices about methods and tools; we also need to make choices about what areas are important enough to spend time tackling. Sustainable improvement takes time and effort, and it is easy to get demoralised if we take on too many projects and can't follow them through. As leaders we have a role to play helping the team to prioritise. We might prefer to do this by instinct, or based on the areas when people seem most enthused. We can also use a more formal process and use a priority matrix, an example of which is shown below. Each area is scored from 1 to 4.

Example of a priority matrix

PROJECT	IMPACT/ IMPORTANCE	WITHIN OUR CONTROL	EASE TO IMPLEMENT	COST/TIME EFFECTIVENESS	SPEED OF IMPLEMENTATION	TOTAL
Reduce broad spectrum antibiotic use	4	4	4	3	3	18
Improve access to appointments	4	3	1	2	1	11
Reduce the number of overdue medication reviews	3	2	2	3	2	12
Increase smear uptake	4	2	2	3	2	13

This can act as a guide on where to start, as the higher scoring areas are most likely to generate improvements.

Over the stile

So far we have been looking at the *why* and the *what* of improvement and the value of gaining a deeper and broader understanding of the current state before getting started on changing things. It's now time to move to *how* to make change happen.

Bibliography

Bowie, P. et al. (2016). Enhancing the effectiveness of significant event analysis: Exploring personal impact and applying systems thinking in primary care. *Journal of Continuing Education in the Health Professions* 36. doi:10.1097/CEH.0000000000000098.

Darzi, A. (2008). *High Quality Care for All.* London, UK: Department of Health.

Gillam, S. & Siriwardena, A.N. (2014). *Quality Improvement in Primary Care: The Essential Guide.* London, UK: Radcliffe.

Ishikawa, K. (1968). *Guide to Quality Control.* Tokyo: JUSE.

Lewin, K. (1951). *Field Theory in Social Science.* New York: Harper and Row.

Lewis, S., Passmore, J., & Cantore, S. (2011). *Appreciative Inquiry for Change Management: Using AI to Facilitate Organizational Development.* London, UK: Kogan-Page.

NHS Improvement. Root Cause Analysis – Using 5 Whys. https://improvement.nhs.uk/documents/2156/root-cause-analysis-five-whys.pdf. Accessed 9 December 2019.

Wiggins, L. & Hunter, H. (2016). *Relational Change: The Art and Practice of Changing Organizations.* London, UK: Bloomsbury Business.

23

Treat improvement like an experiment and measure it

In this chapter, we will explore these questions:

- How can we make improvements happen and make them stick?
- How can we work out how to measure our outcomes to see if our efforts have paid off?
- How can we organise complex change so others can understand what we are doing, and why?

Planning and testing the change

Although it is worth spending time understanding what needs to improve, it is also true that this will keep changing. In the real world of implementing QI, we constantly uncover things we hadn't expected on the journey. Therefore, there will never be a perfect time to get started. Because of the complex, changing context in which we work, there will also never be a perfect solution or endpoint, but QI is a journey of learning and discovery, so the best time to start is probably now.

In healthcare, the most widely recognised method for approaching QI in a structured way is the Institute of Healthcare Improvement's 'model for improvement' (MfI). It is simple and effective and is particularly good for making many sequential small changes that will gradually take us to where we want to be.

The model for improvement – a structured way to plan and test

At the outset, the model for improvement involves answering three questions. In fact, think of it as 'three questions and a wheel', the wheel being a PDSA cycle, which we will explain later in this chapter.

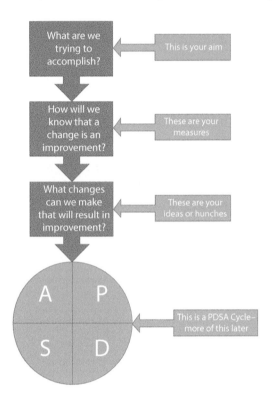

Question 1: what are we trying to accomplish

This question will result in the creation of our 'aim statement'. It sounds very simple, but there is actually quite a knack to it. If this is done well, it can help to focus the project and, lead to better performance. A good aim statement is specific; it includes by how much we want to improve and by when, and is usually worded as a single sentence. Sometimes our aim statements need to include the boundaries of our project, meaning who or what the project is hoping to impact.

Example of setting an aim statement

The doctors and nurses from Jonestown Medical Centre had recently attended a local teaching event on the problems associated with the rise in long-term opioid prescriptions for people for chronic non-malignant pain. They were concerned by what they heard, so they checked out the practice prescribing data and compared it to others in their area. They found that not only were they in the top quarter of prescribers, their prescribing had been steadily increasing over the previous 10 years, despite a stable list size.

Their first step was to set an aim statement.

COMPONENT OF AIM STATEMENT	PRACTICE DECISION
What exactly do we want to improve?	To reduce the number of prescriptions for opioids issued per month
Who is the improvement aimed at?	For patients with chronic non-malignant pain
By how much do we want to improve it?	To be in line with the average number of prescriptions for the locality at the start of the project (which was 50 items/1000 patients/month)
When do we want to have achieved this by?	By two years from the start of the project

Final aim statement: **We will reduce our opioid prescribing for people with chronic non-malignant pain to below 50 items/1000 patients per month by two years from the start of the project.**

By the way we have described this, it might look like the aim statement is set in stone. In the real world of QI where everything is an experiment, we sometimes find we have set the wrong aim. There's not much point in continuing to climb a ladder to the top, if it turns out your ladder is up the wrong wall. Once a QI project is underway, then we start the real learning and can uncover things we hadn't thought of at the outset. This can be particularly true in the complex world of healthcare when the goalposts keep moving. We might uncover other issues that mean we have to make adjustments. In our example, it may be that we have never used a single code for chronic non-malignant pain, making it harder for us to gather our data.

> When the information changes, I change my mind. What do you do?
>
> **John Maynard Keynes**

If new evidence or guidance comes to light suggesting improvement outcomes for patients taking these medications, then clearly the project should take them into account and change if appropriate.

The best aim statement is a SMART one, but at the outset we might not always know if it is. Let's explore this in more depth, using our example above.

Specific	The aim does appear to be specific. However, once the project started, the practice realised they were struggling to know who to exclude. Some patients did have a malignancy, but their opioid had been prescribed for pain not related to this. By excluding them, they felt they were somehow 'cheating' on the project.
Measurable	Because they chose to measure opioids in people without a malignancy, they realised they were relying on staff to be accurate in their coding of diagnoses of malignancy. Once the project started to run, they recognised this coding wasn't as accurate as they had hoped, and it was taking up time manually adjusting the computer searches to get the measures.
Attainable	After the first six months of the project, they realised there were some factors that influenced their prescribing they were struggling to control. They had a rising list size, and many of these patients were transferring from a nearby practice that had the highest opioid prescribing in the locality. Also, the promised holistic pain service that was due to be established locally was delayed, and the practice team found they weren't able to offer the alternatives they had hoped for at the start of the project. They also had failed to recognise the impact of an aging population on their prescribing.
Relevant	The initial aim had included all opioids. As they ran the project, they realised they were successful at reducing prescribing from stronger to weaker opioids, but this improvement wasn't being reflected in their measurements and so they were losing enthusiasm for the project. Their initial aim didn't feel as relevant as it had at the start.
Time-bound	They had set a clear time-frame, but hadn't been able to base this on any other similar projects, and found, in reality, they weren't able to offer the time needed to help people to reduce or stop their opioids in the time frame initially set.

It is easy to become despondent about setting an aim. As we do more QI projects, we get better at setting aims, and find ourselves valuing simplicity over perfection. It may not have mattered about excluding people with malignant pain, as they would be the minority of people on opioids, and the team weren't aiming for zero, so there was plenty of leeway for people with malignant pain to appropriately take opioids. They chose a target that was based on benchmarking data for their locality, but didn't really know if this was achievable or not. An alternative approach might have been to aim for a 5% or 10% reduction in their monthly prescription issues. The purpose for setting a timescale is to keep the momentum up, to help us to plan interventions with enough pace so we can see some change. However, we are constantly challenged by the unpredictable. We need to be agile by being responsive to changing priorities. Something might happen that, quite rightly, pushes our QI project further down the agenda. That's the real world. Alter the timescale ... we are allowed to, as it's OUR project.

Question 2: how will we know that a change is an improvement?

Without data you're just another person with an opinion.

W. Edwards Deming

The second question is about measurements. What exactly will we measure in order to decide if our experiments are working on not? How often will we measure it?

In our experience when teaching QI, talking about measuring can start to reduce the energy in a room. If you love numbers, you may find that data can be very motivating. However, there are factors that can make many of us less enthusiastic about measuring performance, which is often related to previous experience. We will explore them in an attempt to dispel some of the myths around measuring for improvement.

We are constantly judged

In many healthcare systems, we are set targets to achieve related to performance, and often our practice income is dependent on whether we achieve them. In this situation, the data becomes important to our financial sustainability. It is also a pass/fail situation, where the nuances of individual patient variation aren't always appreciated. The targets are set by others, and are generally set in stone meaning we have to manually assess and, if necessary, remove any variations from the target that may be due to an acceptable issue, such as patient preference or a patient's failure to respond to invitations. 'Tidying' the data to ensure that it accurately reflects our performance has become a bureaucratic performance in itself. Understandably, having to do this year on year has made professionals slightly less than excited about data. But this data is gathered for external reasons, for **assurance/accountability.**

QI data is different – it is **our** data, and only we are the people who will be using it to judge **our** projects. It doesn't have to be perfect, or tidy, it just has to be useful.

I was never any good at statistics

Often in our training we learn about research methods: important tools to be able to determine if a medical intervention (drug or procedure) is of real benefit to people or not. We learn about the importance of randomised double-blind placebo controlled trials for therapeutic interventions, controlling for bias in cohort studies and how to calculate and interpret numbers needed to treat, positive predictive values and odds ratios. Unless we are still actively involved in research or in the habit of regularly critically appraising research papers, these skills fade quickly. This is **research data.**

QI data is different – it usually doesn't need you to understand statistics, just be able to follow simple rules.

It's too complicated

Data can often look, and be, very complicated. But it doesn't have to be. Looking back at our experience of general practice data and how it is presented to us over the years tells us where this impression comes from. Supporting GPs, nurses and trainees with clinical audit over the years has shown us that we often make the data complicated ourselves. When conducting an audit we choose too many indicators, and choose indicators that can only be measured by either manually looking through individual patient records, or rely too heavily on, often inaccurate or variable clinical coding. This kind of data is time-consuming to gather, frustrating to interpret and often ineffective at measuring improvement. The other type of data we see is data about how our practice is interacting with the wider health service, such as our referral and admission data. This can sometimes be overwhelming, presented as a spreadsheet and lack any useful guidance on how to interpret it, or how to tell the difference between expected variation and unwarranted variation.

QI data should be different – it needs to be **simple to measure and easy to interpret.**

In summary, data to measure improvement needs to be 'just enough' to tell us if we are improving and frequent enough to tell us if our interventions are having an impact. It is better to choose something simple and easy to measure, that can be done automatically by computer searches rather than manually. If QI work is too time-consuming, motivation often wanes quite quickly.

We will return to explore 'measurement for improvement' later in this chapter.

Question 3: what changes can we make that will result in improvement?

All improvement will require change, but not all change will result in improvement.

G. Langley et al.

In the previous chapter, we shared our thoughts on how to think creatively, both individually and as a group to generate ideas. These skills and techniques are really helpful when coming up with our answer to Question 3 – our change ideas, or our *tests of change.*

This is the fun part. This is when people can contribute their change ideas, things they would like to try out to see what difference they can make. If our teams are already in the habit of sharing their ideas openly without fear or embarrassment, then we don't always have to use any special techniques. In our experience though, practice teams are made up of individuals with a wide range of backgrounds, formal education, and confidence. If we aren't careful, it is always the same people who contribute and we can miss the opportunity of hearing the ideas of those less used to, or comfortable in speaking out. Special engagement and facilitation techniques can be very helpful to bring out the ideas of a wider group of people.

Example

Practice X decided they would like to improve their cervical screening uptake, which had fallen below the national target figure for the first time in years. They set their aim statement and their measures.

Jane, the practice manager, decided to facilitate a meeting of GPs, practice nurses and reception staff to come up with some ideas for change. One of the practice nurses, Moira, had been the practice lead on the smear programme for years and had previously done this in isolation. Jane felt that harnessing the ideas of the whole team might help them think of things they hadn't tried before, but at the same time was concerned everyone would stay quiet as they had got into the habit of leaving everything related to smears to Moira.

Jane started the meeting by reminding everyone of the aim statement and why the project had been chosen. She set the purpose of the meeting as being specifically about ideas generation, and asked everyone the think as creatively as they could, considering things that may never have been tried before.

There were 12 people at the meeting, with varied roles in the practice. Jane paired up the participants, being careful not to pair a louder member of the team with a quieter member, to ensure that the quieter voices were heard. To stimulate their deeper thinking, she asked them to think about when they were last called up for any kind of screening tests or check-up (for example their own smear, dental check-up or other health screening). She asked them to have a 5-minute conversation about what factors affected whether they went for the test or not. They were also given permission to broaden the conversation to consider people they knew, and what had affected their decision to attend. She asked the pairs to write what they had thought of on a piece of paper.

After the 5-minute conversation, she asked them to read over the factors on their list and, by considering these, come up with two ideas that would have made them, or others, more likely to book an appointment for a smear. Each idea was then written on a Post-it note and passed to Jane.

Ideas generated are shown in the illustration.

Create a reminder from the practice instead of just from the National screening programme	Tell a 'patient story' on the waiting room TV Information screen	Create an alert on the medical records so reception team can prompt women to book in
Put a message on the Waiting Room check-in screen prompting women 25–64 years old to ask reception when they last had a smear	Set up some smear information display boards using different languages	Tell a 'patient story' on the Practice facebook page. Consider a patient from an ethnic group with low uptake.
Phone women who have never had a smear to see what the reasons are	Thank you letter given to women after their smear, asking them to encourage their friends to come	Create more smear appointment slots before and after normal working hours
Invites to include information on how to book a smear out of normal working hours	Text reminders for smear appointments to day before	Send text saying 'thank you for booking your smear' after appointment has been made

Once the ideas had all been collected, they were stuck on to the meeting room whiteboard and grouped according to theme. Jane was really pleased about how much energy and enthusiasm there was amongst the reception team for helping to solve the issue. Moira was relieved to finally have some help and support. The next step was to prioritise which idea to try out first.

A shared exercise to generate ideas can result in two outcomes. Not only do we generate ideas for testing, but we also influence the team dynamic and the organisational culture. A difficult issue becomes a shared issue. When we have been involved in generating change ideas, we are then more likely to actively participate in implementing them. This is particularly important when we have to change our own behaviour, for example when we need to start responding to alerts that we may previously have ignored. In the example above, delegating all the responsibility for all things related to smears to the practice nurse was part of the organisational culture; it was 'how we always do things round here'. The 30-minute meeting to generate change ideas went a long way to alter this culture to one where teamwork was valued and people felt a sense of shared responsibility.

Top tip

Try to avoid lifting change ideas from other sources (such as from the examples in this book) but actually go through the process of generating them as a team. Even if you end up with the same change ideas, you are unlikely to end up with the same engagement in implementing them.

Which idea do we test out first?

If we were to take a purist QI approach, then we would always test out one change idea at a time, to see which makes the most difference to the outcome. This way we can ensure that the change is embedded and sustained in the longer term, and we don't waste resources continuing with changes that don't work. However, in reality, especially if we have generated energy around a project and if some of the changes are simple and easy to implement, we often find multiple new things occur at the same time and it is hard to know which have generated the most difference. This doesn't always have to matter, as crushing people's enthusiasm may be more detrimental to our desired 'culture of improvement' than know exactly which intervention works. A skilled leader walks the tight rope between methodology and engagement and gets successfully to the other side.

If we do decide to do more systematic tests of change, then we need to decide which change to test first. As leaders of change we could choose to do this in a random way, just following where the energy seems greatest or we could decide to be more systematic. It's clear there are advantages and disadvantages of each approach, and we will have our own natural styles of approaching these things.

ADVANTAGES OF NOT HAVING A STRICT PLAN	ADVANTAGES OF A SYSTEMATIC APPROACH
Can be energising and maintain people's enthusiasm	First changes are the ones most likely to make a difference
The easiest changes are usually made first so can be resource efficient	Prevents the change being dominated by those individuals with the loudest voices
Changes implemented more quickly	Changes implemented more effectively

One systematic way of discovering which change to try first is to gather some data about the problem area to help us decide. Earlier in this chapter, we described eight tools for unpicking and exploring issues more deeply. If we have already used some of the methods described, this may have given us a steer on which idea to try out first. It can be very helpful to quantify this using a Pareto chart, which helps our team to visualise the issues causing a problem in order to prioritise our response.

Example of using a Pareto chart

The staff at Practice Y were disappointed when they saw the results from a national audit of care of people with diabetes. Only 42% of their patients with diabetes had had all of the recommended 'processes of care' in the last 12 months. When they looked more closely at the results, they could see the area they fell down on was recording patient's body mass index (BMI).

They discussed this at a practice meeting and the team could think of several reasons why BMI wasn't being recorded.

They decided to do review some case notes to find out which intervention might be the most useful. They looked at 30 patients with diabetes who had not had their BMI recorded in the last 12 months to figure out the reason.

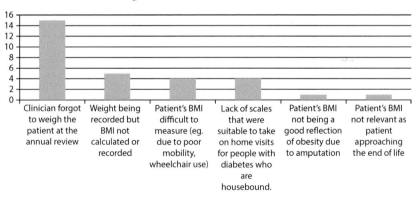

As a result of the Pareto chart, they decided to look for ideas to make it easier for the clinician to remember to weigh the patient at their annual review, such as a prompt put on the records.

We will never live in a perfect world, and aiming for 100% coverage with any intervention can actually lead to inappropriate activity, such as weighing people who are terminally ill for the purposes of 'preventive' care.

Pareto charts are useful for gaining a bit of perspective. We often only need to try to solve the two or three most frequent problems in order to generate big gains.

If our ideas aren't as easy to measure as those in the example above, we can prioritise them using other criteria. We might decide to rank them in order of how easy they might be to implement, or by how many resources (time and money) might be needed to implement them. It can also be helpful to use a voting system.

Example of a voting system to prioritise change ideas – back to Practice X's Smear Uptake Project

Lots of ideas had been generated and at the next practice meeting, Jane, the practice manager, planned an exercise to prioritise the ideas. She wrote each idea on a piece of A4 paper and stuck them around the walls of the meeting room.

Each member of staff was given two sticky dots and were asked to place them on the idea they liked best, taking into consideration how likely they felt it would be effective and how much resource would be taken up implementing it.

At the end of the exercise the ideas were ranked in order according to how many dots they had acquired. The ranking then triggered a conversation as to whether this had generated an appropriate order.

Time to start testing: how to use PDSA cycles

Once we have decided on our ideas for testing, each idea gets plugged into something called a PDSA cycle. This stands for 'Plan Do Study Act'. Good leadership helps the whole process by encouraging experimentation, changing attitudes to failing (because we learn, there is no such thing as actually failing) and depersonalising the process of change through the use of data.

Plan Start with one of the change ideas. Remember to start small; it's a steady climb, not a pole vault.

- Work out the practical steps needed to make it happen (Who? When? How? Where?).

- Make sure that we have predicted what we are hoping will happen and have identified something relevant that we can measure.

- Work out what we need to look out for that might mean our change is causing unintended harm, for example, if we are trying to reduce antibiotic prescribing, is our admission rate for infections increasing?

Do Let's try it

- Carry out the plan
- Make a note of any problems
- Begin measuring whatever we decided would be a good measure of success

Study Did it work?

- Look at the data; display it in a chart rather than a table so that everyone can understand it
- Compare results to the predictions
- Consider the qualitative results (how did it feel?) as well as the numbers
- Work out if the results have shown success. Don't worry if they haven't, at least you will have learned something. 'Fail fast to improve quickly'.
- Check out the problem areas, as the risks may need to be mitigated in future cycles.

Act What's next?

- Based on the results, decide if it is enough to continue the same intervention, or will we need to add something else to get to our goal? It would be rare to achieve absolute success with the first cycle. It is more likely you discover something that needs adjusting before it reliably achieves what we are hoping for.
- Adjust, adapt or choose a new intervention. Then start the cycle again.

Some practices and organisations are dynamic and agile and find implementing improvement is a natural part of how they operate. In this situation, they are often continuously implementing PDSA cycles, without necessarily being aware this is what they are doing. The process doesn't have to be complex and onerous. In fact, it shouldn't be.

Involving patients in the planning of our projects can bring new insights that can influence their success. In the previous section *What needs to improve?* we discussed ways of involving patients and carers in working out our improvement needs. They can also help us plan and implement projects.

Example of involving patients in planning

> Practice X had decided to attempt a reduction in opioid prescribing and their first idea for testing was a letter to patients explaining the possible harm of long-term opioid use and inviting them to discuss a reduction plan with their doctor. Dr A drafted a letter and asked one of her patients, Rita, who had been taking tramadol for many years for back pain, for an honest opinion on the letter. Dr A was surprised when Rita said she found the letter quite judgmental and that she felt like a 'drug addict' after reading it. Together they reworded the letter until both were happy with the new version.

Looking out for unintended consequences is an important part of any QI project. For example, in a project to reduce the number of times patients miss appointments, doctors and nurses may start to run late or feel more stressed. These missed appointments are sometimes used as valuable 'catch up' time. Knowing this might mean we still plan the intervention but reduce the number of bookable appointments to allow for a higher attendance rate.

Teams typically have some members who are particularly good at spotting what might go wrong with a project. People with this skill might have been considered to be a barrier to change, with a tendency to say 'Yes, but ...' whenever as change idea is suggested. They don't have to be a barrier; instead their skill can be put to good use, making predictions of things to watch out for.

One practice we worked with decided they would like to open up their Saturday flu immunisation clinic to online booking. After thinking about this, the practice IT manager said 'Yes, but people might book a slot when they aren't eligible for an NHS flu jab'. They were aware that every year there were a handful of people who were immunised without being in a 'target group', so it was reasonable to be concerned this might increase if the appointments were available for people to book without going through the 'filter' of a reception phone call. So, the practice decided to check for this. After the first 50 appointments had been booked, they checked if there was any difference in the rate of inappropriate bookings between those appointments that had been booked by phone and those booked online. They were happy to report no increase in inappropriate booking so felt confident to continue the intervention.

Data for improvement

This section will not attempt to be a comprehensive guide to measuring quality improvement in healthcare. There are many excellent resources on this topic. Instead, we will describe the principles and describe some of the tools we have found most useful in a primary care setting. Analysing data is an important part of the 'Study' in our PDSA cycles.

Data principle 1: Gather it frequently

The QI is a dynamic process, and we rarely achieve success with our first intervention (or 'test of change'). Gathering data little and often will tell us if our interventions are working.

Data principle 2: Display it well, over time

Data displayed in a table is hard to make sense of. If our data is always displayed visually and over time, we can see which of our interventions have made the most difference and can look back to see how far we have come. Over the last few years, hospital wards that are involved in QI work often use display boards on the ward to show staff, patients, and visitors how they are performing against areas they are aiming to improve. In a similar way, general practice performance boards, as a place to display our data can help to remind us of projects we are working on, generate discussion and also motivate us when we have successes to share.

Example of data display

The proportion of women who book their smear after receiving an invitation, per month.

YEAR 1		YEAR 2	
January	0.7	January	0.74
February	0.72	February	0.77
March	0.65	March	0.77
April	0.82	April	0.78
May	0.74	May	0.76
June	0.78	June	0.81
July	0.68	July	0.82
August	0.72	August	0.79
September	0.74	September	0.81
October	0.7	October	0.84
November	0.78	November	0.81
December	0.73	December	0.85

When displayed in a tabular format it's really hard for anyone to tell what is really happening. If the same data is displayed in a chart, the real impact of our improvement interventions becomes clear:

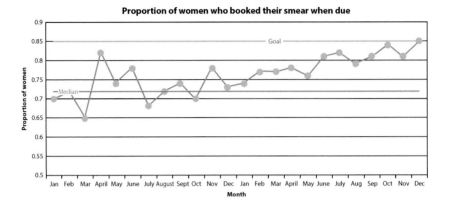

Proportion of women who booked their smear when due

Data principle 3: Understand variable data

The simplest way of measuring our success is by using 'before and after' measurements. By this we mean looking at the data before we make our change and then again afterwards. Unfortunately, if we do this, we might fail to pick up on whether the change is **real** or not, especially if the data varies from week to week or month to month, just in line with normal variations in our day to day work.

The following illustration is an example of why this is important. It shows data from a project to reduce the number of minutes each patient spends waiting before they are called in for their appointment. Just looking at the 'before and after' data on the left makes the project seem more successful than it really was.

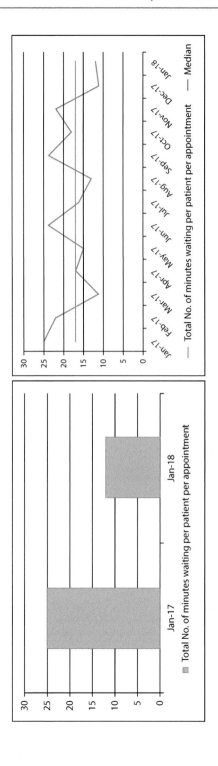

The chart to the right is an example of a *run chart*. This is a graph of our data on the *y*-axis, against time on the *x*-axis, with the median of all the data points drawn as the horizontal line. The data crosses the median line frequently, and this shows that there is a natural variation in performance that we hadn't previously appreciated. The variation in waiting time is likely to relate to things such as case mix, clinician fatigue, IT performance, and so on. This is known as *common cause variation*. If the thing we have chosen to measure in our QI project is likely to be something variable, like monthly issues of opioid prescriptions, for example, then we need to gather baseline data, ideally for 15 data points, so that we can understand the variability before we start to test out our change ideas. Sometimes this means we need to delay the start of our project, though more often we can collect the baseline data retrospectively.

Once we have our baseline data, we fix the median, make our changes and then continue to gather the data to see what happens. In order to see if there has been an improvement we will be looking to see if there is a shift, or a trend in the new data, compared with the baseline.

A shift is when six or more of the new data points consecutively fall to one side or the other of the median–showing you have made a change. This data shows a shift downwards.

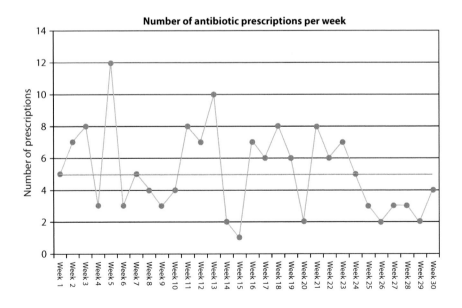

Number of antibiotic prescriptions per week

A trend is when five or more of the new data points go sequentially upwards or downwards. This data shows a trend downwards.

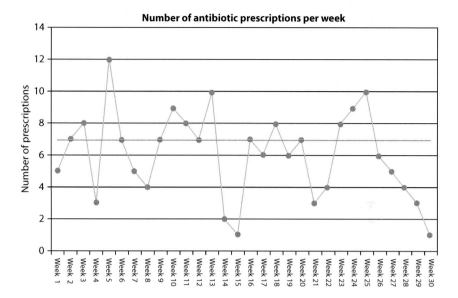

Data principle 4: Know how to set control lines once your data is stable to ensure that quality is sustained

In certain situations, when we have achieved a new level of performance, we want to continue measuring to check to see if the performance is sustained. In this situation, we need to know if our variation is falling within statistically expected variability. This is when *Statistical Process Control (SPC) Charts* can be useful.

An SPC chart is a method for displaying performance data to check if the performance is continuing to be as expected. They are a better option than run charts for identifying 'freak' points above or below the majority of the data points as they use the mean for their centre line. This approach makes 'freak' points stand out, giving a clear signal that something unusual has happened. This is known as 'special cause variation'.

The SPC charts include 'control lines' above and below the mean, which tell us when our process may be starting to perform in an unexpected way. Control lines (or limits) are created by using the data we have gathered about our system and its performance using our run chart. The standard deviation of the data is calculated and the lines are drawn at values that would represent 3 SDs either side of the mean, one line above (the 'upper control limit'), and one line below (the 'lower control limit'). This means that at least 99% of all future data would be expected to fall between these two control lines.

If a data point is outside of the upper or lower control limits (<99% likelihood that this has happened by chance), this is either a concern to be investigated, or a sign that our intervention is making a difference.

Example of an SPC chart

This chart shows the number of days patients would need to wait until the next appointment for ear syringing. The practice was happy with their mean of just over 12 days, as this left time for the wax softening drops to work. They set 'control limits' on the chart, which showed that on one occasion the wait time was longer than what was expected by normal (or 'common cause') variation. They realised this was because a clinic had been cancelled due to a training day. When reviewing the data they decided to add an additional clinic whenever clinics were cancelled.

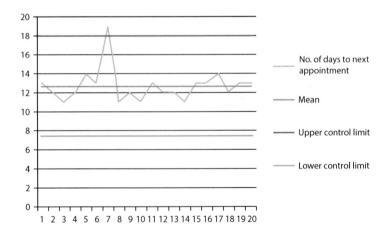

Different types of data (e.g., continuous or discrete) require different mathematical techniques to create the SPC chart, and statistical packages can be bought to help with this.

In a GP practice there are few systems and processes that warrant using SPC charts. However, as GPs work more 'at scale' there are likely to be more opportunities to use this type of chart to analyse system performance to check out for unexpected changes.

Organising quality improvement: driver diagrams

Sometimes the area we want to improve can seem so complex and generates such a breadth of change ideas it feels overwhelming. It is easy to lose sight of both the overall aim, and how each change is designed to drive the improvement we want. In this situation, a *driver diagram* can help us organise and display our improvement strategy in a logical way, to clearly explain our 'theory of change'. The diagram is focused around a single clear improvement aim, though some organisations use a driver diagram to plan the direction of their work following development of a vision or mission statement. There are four levels to a driver diagram:

- The **'aim'** is what we are trying to achieve, which ideally is something measurable. This will usually be the statement we created when answering the first question from the model for improvement.
- The **'primary drivers'** are a set of broad areas on which we need to work in order to achieve our aim.
- The **'secondary drivers'** are the more specific areas of work that influence our primary drivers. Each primary driver will be influenced by several secondary drivers. Secondary drivers may impact on more than one primary driver.
- **'Change ideas'** are generated by the team.

When completed, the diagram provides a change strategy that can be shared and understood, and provides the basis for planning the individual projects or interventions. It should not be considered 'fixed', and can change over time as improvements are generated. Using a driver diagram means that instead of coming up with random ideas or favouring ones suggested by people with power, we can generate logical ideas we know could have an impact on the aim.

Example of creating a driver diagram

The team at Practice Z were finding they seemed to be working harder and harder to keep up with day-to-day patient requests for care. They had spent an 'away day' exploring the issues and decided they may be able to reduce some of their workload by developing more efficient systems to managing the incoming demand. They identified many reasons for the increasing demand for same day services and ideas for change and so decided to create a driver diagram to organise their thinking. This was then displayed in the meeting room and they came back to it monthly to track how they were doing with the project.

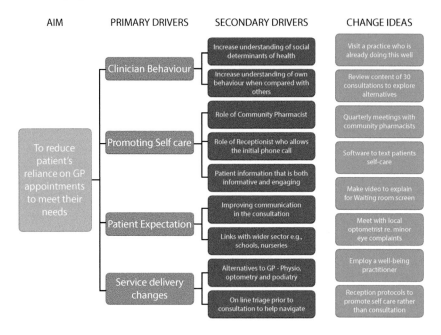

Improving the system

It is clear that all improvements require change, but not all changes will result in improvement. If we take an issue such as a sudden increase in demand for GP appointments, we might treat it in one of two ways. We might mistake it as a blip rather than as a system problem and therefore choose to do nothing about it. Alternatively, we may think the problem is due to something fundamental and seek to change the whole system when actually it's a blip (e.g., a couple of staff on holiday) and a short-term fix would have been appropriate.

Changes in one part of the system can produce predicted changes elsewhere (which is what we hope for) but also unpredicted changes in other parts of the system or at a later time. These unintended consequences are common and can lead to misinterpretation of the causes, so we need to beware.

We have a natural tendency, when problems occur, to assume that it is *people* who are to blame rather than the system itself. Generally speaking, we have bad systems (which can include staff training) rather than bad people.

To build up evidence of whether changes do result in improvement, it is often better to give resources to the early adopters and enthusiasts rather than wait for everyone to come on board. Be careful not to let 'perfect' be the enemy of 'good'. Sometimes, in the hunt for the perfect intervention, we just delay matters; instead try a series of small tests and learn sequentially from them.

The whole purpose of testing is that it increases people's *belief* in the changes that are being made. It does this if two conditions are met:

- The predictions that we made about what the intervention could achieve, are supported by the evidence.

- The conditions under which the evidence was obtained are roughly similar to the conditions on which the prediction was based.

By getting people involved in the intervention and the analysis, they help to create a new system. People tend to support systems they help to create.

Beneficial changes result in the creation of a structure that makes it easy for people to do the right thing (use the new system) and hard to do the wrong thing (go back to the old system). For example, if we brought in a template system for generating referral letters, we might design a simple link from the patient's notes to the template and simultaneously, remove the old system of dictating referral letters.

It can be understandably tempting to speed things up by automating the system. However, we should resist doing this until we know that what we are automating is the right or best way of dealing with an issue. If we don't pause to take this step, we may end up making it even easier to do the wrong thing.

So many of our leadership activities relate to making improvements to systems, processes, and outcomes for our patients and our teams. Quality improvement is likely to play a significant part in our leadership hike. Taking a systematic QI approach can give us a framework, or map to use, that can help us to navigate through the complexities. Using this map, we can engage our teams in the work and generate some meaningful data to demonstrate what difference we are making.

Over the stile

The last three chapters have detailed a range of QI tools and methods to help us deliver better care for our patients and a better workplace for our teams. However, it isn't the tools and methods that make things better, it is always the people, and people often find change really hard. In the next chapter, we will move into the area of managing change, including the human psychological response to change, and explore different change models that can act as a lens to use when choosing the right approach.

Bibliography

Carey, R.G. & Lloyd, R.C. (1995). *Measuring Quality Improvement in Healthcare*. New York, NY: ASQ Quality Press.

Langley, G.J. et al. (2009). *The Improvement Guide: A Practical Approach to Enhancing Organizational Performance* (2nd ed.). San Francisco, CA: Jossey-Bass. ISBN: 978-0-470-19241-2.

24

Change and how to manage it

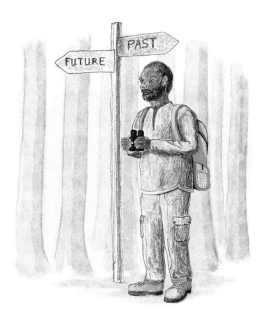

- Why do people appear to find change difficult?
- How can we make it easier for all?
- When should we plan change, and when should we just aim to create the right environment to make it happen?

All improvement involves change. Change is an inevitable part of our lives, as well as our work. As leaders it can be useful to explore some theoretical change models to help us make sense of how people around us are responding to change. In this section, we explore both leading change, and managing change. In Chapter 2, we described some features of leadership and management. Managing change effectively needs us to be skilled in both.

As well as exploring types of change, this section will describe some models used by leaders to help them facilitate change. The previous section explored the principles and some of the tools used in quality improvement (QI). Here, we will look at change from a more planned, strategic perspective, rather than the 'ground up' approach usually used for QI. This can be a more appropriate way of organising a complicated service development such as establishing a primary care network, or the merger of a group of practices. Here, we will mostly keep our focus on the significant issues at practice level. We will look at the people and the psychology of change, how we might analyse why and where things go wrong and how we can project-manage within a complex system.

Why change?

Both external and internal forces drive changes to our practice. We live in an ever-changing world and our practices operate within a complex wider system of health and social care, which is influenced by changes in political ideology, changes to funding structures and contracts and alterations in population expectations and needs. Much of this is out of our control. Change is how we adapt and evolve in order to continue to do the job we love and deliver the care we feel our populations deserve within the limits of our resources.

But change is difficult as it often involves losing something as we transition to a new way of working. If we learn to recognise what is being lost, it will help us to lead others more successfully through the change.

The psychological dimensions of change

Why before what

For things to change, it usually means people have to change. Most primary care professionals have a certain amount of understanding of behavioural change and motivational interviewing. We do this with our patients frequently, trying to work out where they are up to in their personal 'cycle of change' and how ready they are to make that leap into the great unknown of more exercise, less alcohol or fewer cigarettes. We covered human motivation and how to influence it in Chapter 14. Similar principles apply when we are trying to lead people through a service change, or change to their working habits or behaviours. Some people just need to be told what to do and they do it, but they are rare. Most of us need to know why we are doing it. Business guru Simon Sinek has sold millions of books focussing mainly on this fact: 'The WHY is the purpose, cause or belief that drives every one of us'.

If we understand why we are doing something, it helps us to deliver it more effectively. If we can help others to understand and accept this too, we can influence how they behave, and change will happen.

Transitions

With change comes loss, and this is often the reason we find it so difficult. Bridges, an organisational change expert wrote extensively on this in his book *Managing Transitions*. He made a distinction between change and transition: 'Change is situational: the move to a new site, the retirement of the founder, the reorganisation of the roles on the team, the revisions to the pension plan. Transition, on the other hand, is psychological; it is a three-phase process that people go through as they internalise and come to terms with the details of the new situation that the change brings about'.

In Chapter 3, we described what it means to be courageous. A transition is an extended phase of being courageous, both individually and collectively. If we can recognise which phase we, our team, or the individuals within the team are at in the transition process, it helps us choose the right approach that helps change to happen more smoothly.

Phase 1: Ending, losing, letting go

We enter this as soon as the change is mentioned. The change is likely to involve leaving the current state. Even if the current state is not great, the new state is unknown and potentially threatening and uncomfortable. We may not have fully understood how important some roles or tasks are to the people who carry them out. During this phase, people feel fear, denial, sadness, confusion, and uncertainty. It is important not to argue too hard for the change, although at the same time, frequently remind people gently of the 'Why'. Accept some resistance as inevitable, legitimise the emotions the change engenders and listen with empathy. Communicate openly and frequently, and give people a clear idea of what they will be doing in the 'new state'. Be patient.

Phase 2: The neutral zone

> One doesn't discover new lands without consenting to lose sight of the shore for a very long time.
>
> **André Gide, French Novelist**

Some changes take a long time to implement and get right (see the example below). This can mean a long time spent 'in the wilderness' between the old state and the new, when no one really knows what is happening. It can feel akin to letting go of a trapeze without being sure the next trapeze is going to appear for you to grasp. During this phase people can feel anxious, resentful, sceptical, and impatient. We might find the practice is less productive during this phase. We can help people through this phase by reassurance and giving a sense of direction where possible, for example, by setting short-term goals to show the project is on track. Encourage people and celebrate even small successes.

Phase 3: Launching a new beginning

During this phase, people may feel re-energised and optimistic. They are becoming more familiar with their new role or system and are learning new competencies and can see the opportunities this may bring. This isn't an inevitable phase; some people can get stuck in the previous phases and people move through the phases at different rates. As leaders we can help by continuing with the encouragement and reinforcing the successes. It can be helpful to look back at how far we have come and to see this change in the context of the long-term 'story' of the organisation. Celebrate all the hard work it has taken to get to the end.

One of the most difficult changes we can remember during our working life was the switch over to a new electronic medical record system. The picture captures some of the conversations that occurred placed in the context of Bridge's transition phases.

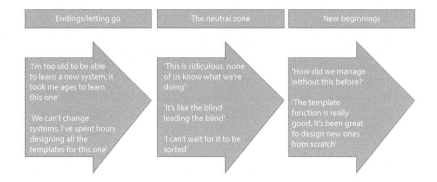

An awareness of this transition process can help build our confidence as leaders; accepting the negative reaction as part of a normal process helps us be patient and to maintain our own sense of well-being through the process. It also means we are more likely to welcome conversations about the change, rather than avoid them. It's keeping the conversations going that will help us all through transitions.

Types of organisational change

Business experts and researchers describe a wide range of change models that fall loosely into two groups:

* Planned, structured or directive change
* Emergent, facilitative or relational change

We feel there is a role for both, and that an awareness of which approach we are using, plus an ability to adapt our approach depending on the circumstances helps us lead change more effectively. Even if we decide to use an emergent change model, there will be elements that are more stable and predictable and allow for a more planned approach.

Planned change

A well-known structural approach to change was proposed by John Kotter. His model consists of eight steps, although he acknowledges that each step may need to be revisited during the change process.

1 *Establish a sense of urgency*
    To provide momentum for the change (create a 'burning platform')

2 *Create a guiding coalition*
    Including people with the power to lead the change

3 *Develop a vision and strategy*
    To help direct the change effort

4 *Communicate the change vision*
    As widely as possible, and leaders to model the change

5 *Empower broad-based action*
    Get rid of obstacles, change systems and structures, encourage all involved

6 *Generate short-term wins*
    Quick wins to motivate, recognise those who made them possible

7 *Consolidate gains to produce more change*
    This may mean engaging with more people

8 *Embed the new approaches in the culture*
    The change is no longer a project, but 'the way we do things'

Although we can see how attractive it is to see leading change in this way, the model has been criticised for focussing more on the actions of the leader in 'driving' the change and less on the importance of relationships and influencing human behaviours in generating change. Rather than seeing Kotter as a stepwise model for managing change, it can be useful to use it as a lens to explore why change attempts fail, for example, by not recognising the importance of particular elements, such as creating a coalition that includes those who have the power to stand in the way. Alternatively, failing to look ahead and plan to deliver some quick wins in order to maintain motivation, which predictably dips shortly after the initial enthusiasm that people feel at the start of a project.

Another tool often used in a process of planned change is an 'options appraisal', through which a number of potential options for action are evaluated and preferred courses of action are identified.

Example of an options appraisal

Practice C was undecided on what to do following the retirement of their senior partner. They were aware that other practices in the neighbourhood had vacancies that they were struggling to fill. They conducted a basic options appraisal.

	BENEFITS	RISK	COST	UNCERTAINTIES
Option 1 **Do nothing**	No upheaval	Stress to remaining GPs due to high workload Longer wait times for patients	Higher income for remaining partners Remaining partners have to take out a loan to buy out senior partner	Not sure how much it may cost in locums
Option 2 **Try to recruit a new partner**	Familiar model, know what to expect Can buy out leaving partner	May take a long time to recruit Inflexible if circumstances change	Cost neutral, other than legal expenses for new partnership agreement	Future of structure of primary care uncertain
Option 3 **Try to recruit a salaried GP**	Flexible, can give notice if practice circumstances change	May take a long time to recruit May not remain in post long	Remaining partners have to take out a loan to buy out senior partner	Uncertain if we will find someone suitable
Option 4 **Recruit an Advanced Nurse Practitioner (ANP)**	Better skill mix as ANP trained in managing same day demand leaving more GP time for complex care Flexible, can give notice if practice circumstances change Opportunity to discover what other roles can offer the practice	May not stay in post long, ANPs currently moving from practice to practice	Cheaper hourly rate than a GP Remaining partners have to take out a loan to buy out senior partner	Not sure what an ANP can deliver

(*Continued*)

	BENEFITS	RISK	COST	UNCERTAINTIES
Option 5 **Become a training practice**	New GPs coming through the practice meaning it may be easier to recruit in future Career development for existing GP to be a trainer	Patients will have to see a range of new GPs, affecting continuity Inexperienced GPs Lots of time taken in achieving the standards needed to be a training practice	Cheapest option as salary not paid by practice Remaining partners have to take out a loan to buy out senior partner	How much time it will take for the trainer

The exercise led to them deciding to visit a neighbouring practice that was employing an ANP to see what they offered the practice, as this looked like the most viable option.

Following the decision about an intended course of action, we can develop a detailed plan on how to implement the change. The final section of this chapter describes some project techniques and a tool that can support us with this. This planned approach to change can be quite comforting. It helps us to feel assured that we haven't forgotten anything important, which is especially helpful when the process seems complicated. It lends itself well to a series of checklists and checkpoints to ensure we are on track. As a leader of this type of change, we will find ourselves being fairly directive; telling our team what needs to happen and by when. This can also be a comfort to our team to know what is expected of them. In Chapter 1, we explored the difference between issues that are simple, complicated, and complex. A planned approach to change can be helpful with complicated changes (rather than complex); when we are fairly certain about the solution to our issue, and there is a high degree of agreement across the team that this is the right thing to do.

Emergent/facilitative change

In Chapter 1, we defined the health care environment as a complex adaptive system with multiple parts. Even having a good understanding of how all the individual components behave doesn't always help us predict how the whole system will interact to generate outcomes. Let's get a feel for the complex world we inhabit.

Probably, no other healthcare sector has so many complex parts – such elaborate funding models, the multiple services that vary according to geography, and so many options and interventions for any one person's needs. Patient presentation is uncertain and unique, and there are many options for investigation and action that must be individualised to each patient, allowing for their preference and need. Alongside this there are numerous stakeholders, with different roles and interests, and inconsistent regulations that tightly control some matters and barely touch others. In this environment, it seems unlikely we will ever have a high amount of agreement or certainty about which change will be right to achieve the outcome we want.

It wouldn't be surprising if, as we gain better awareness about the complexity of our leadership journey, we start to feel anxious. How could anyone be expected to effectively lead change under these circumstances?

Understanding and adopting a model of emergent change can help us find our way through this. An emergent change model embraces the concept that we may not know the answer in advance, and instead creates the right environment for positive change to emerge, often in unpredictable ways.

So, what is the right environment, and how do we, as leaders create it? Human beings are by nature social animals. We are influenced so much by what is going around us, by trends and by conversations we have. Chapter 9 has explored in depth the importance and barriers to effective dialogue. In a complex world, change can happen through conversations where both parties are striving to understand each other. Creating opportunities for conversations can be one of our most important leadership acts. In the busy world of general practice and primary care it is easier to send an email in place of arranging a conversation, but an email will very rarely achieve the same outcome. We can create policy, protocols and rules that are written and ratified, but no one follows; and yet we find that people can change the way they do things sometimes just following a single conversation.

Finding ways to make sure everyone has a clear understanding of, and ideally shares the overall vision for the practice or organisation (see Chapter 17) helps positive change to emerge from the conversations, as does paying attention to the factors influencing our practice culture, particularly if these factors get in the way of people connecting authentically with each other.

The advantage of taking a more facilitative approach to change is the flexibility that it brings when we encounter factors we weren't expecting.

The best-laid plans of mice and men often go awry.

Adapted from Robert Burns

Although within this process there will be phases of stability that can be managed using linear approaches, extreme adherence to a linear plan can mean that we become blinkered to the possibility our plan may be wrong. The traditional model of the charismatic leader with a clear vision they 'drive forward' heavily relies on the vision being the right one. Taking a more facilitative or relational approach to change takes the pressure off the leader to be right and opens up possibilities beyond those that had been originally planned.

Project management

At times practices suffer from 'too much leadership and not enough management'. In these organisations, the culture is often dynamic and exciting, with a clear vision and purpose. Change is welcomed and there are opportunities for the type of conversations that help change to happen. Sounds like a great place to work? But if there isn't enough management of projects, things become chaotic, important issues are forgotten and risks emerge, which can be both clinical and financial. The GPs and practice managers may have never had any formal training in project management and may have been making it up as they go along, albeit sometimes very effectively.

The project management process

If we take a step-by-step approach to project management then these steps have proved useful:

1 Agree precise specification for the project
2 Decide who is going to be involved (the project team)
3 Communicate the project plan to your project team – and to any other interested people and groups
4 Set meeting dates/times
5 Plan the project – create a check list of tasks, budget and possible risks. Plan the times scales and consider using a Gantt chart (see below)
6 Agree and delegate project tasks
7 Manage and motivate – inform, encourage and enable the project team
8 Check, measure, monitor, review project progress – adjust project plans, and inform the project team and others

9 Complete project – review and report on project performance; celebrate success

10 Project follow-up – train, support, measure and report results and benefits

Gantt charts

Gantt charts are useful project management tools. They are named after the US engineer and consultant Henry Gantt, who devised the technique in the 1910s. Simply put, a Gantt chart is a visual view of tasks scheduled over time. The charts are used for planning and tracking projects as they show which task in the project is scheduled to be done over which time period. They also help us see the start and end dates of a project in one simple view.

The example below is a Gantt chart showing a project to employ a new member of staff, showing this as a 7-month project that starts at the advertisement and finishes with the new team member's 3-month appraisal. More complex projects lead to more complex charts, with the tasks subdivided into overall headings, or pertaining to different sub-groups involved in the implementation of the project.

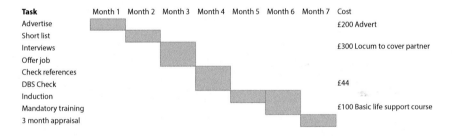

Task	Month 1	Month 2	Month 3	Month 4	Month 5	Month 6	Month 7	Cost
Advertise								£200 Advert
Short list								
Interviews								£300 Locum to cover partner
Offer job								
Check references								
DBS Check								£44
Induction								
Mandatory training								£100 Basic life support course
3 month appraisal								

This example was created with a basic knowledge of Excel, although more sophisticated Gantt chart software (or equivalent) is available online.

Risk management

Pretty much every project we implement carries some degree of risk. Recognising the possible risks in advance helps us look out for them and take steps to reduce the risk. Even the employment of a new member of staff risks us choosing the wrong person, or choosing the right person but them dropping out before the start date. Other projects may carry risks related to the care we provide our patients. For example, when one practice installed a new telephone system which included voice mail facilities, it failed to recognise that callers leaving long messages on voice mails tied up the incoming phone lines meaning many more people failed to get through. Recognising this as a risk in advance could have led to a more gradual testing process and avoided three days of long queues of angry patients at the reception desk. Recognising risk in advance often takes the 'sting' out of it when it happens, allowing us a more measured response and reducing stress.

Over the stile

Leading and managing change is as much about managing your interactions with people as it is understanding the principles of project management. Although having some structure to how we lead change and manage projects can provide security and minimise risk, it is managing the relational and psychological aspects of change that our leadership skills are most needed and provide our chance to shine. We need to be mindful not to let our plan cloud our vision or limit our adaptability.

We are now moving to the final leg of our leadership journey. In Chapter 6, we explore the additional challenges faced by senior leaders, and the skills we need to lead beyond our usual boundaries where there may be opportunities to make a significant difference to the health of the population that we serve.

Bibliography

Bridges, W. (2017). *Managing Transitions: Making the Most of Change* (4th ed.). London, UK: Nicholas Brealey Publishing. ISBN-10: 1473664500.

Kotter, J. (2012). *Leading Change.* Harvard Business Review. ISBN-10: 9781422186435.

Sinek, S. (2011). *Start With Why: How Great Leaders Inspire Everyone to Take Action.* London, UK: Penguin. ISBN-10: 9780241958223.

6

A view from the top: A wider horizon

Section introduction

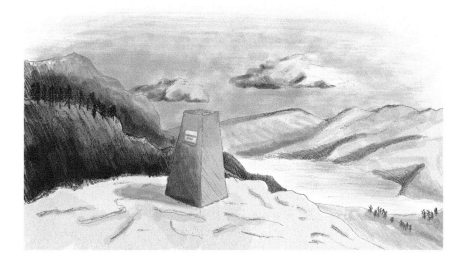

It's been a long journey, but we have learned a great deal about ourselves and about the people with whom we work. Through this, we can become highly effective leaders within our practices and local communities, and for many leaders that will be more than enough. However, it is the nature of climbing that the higher we go, the further we can often see. We should be open to the possibility that as our perspective changes, so may our ambition for what can be done.

We have reached a point in our journey where we have significant leadership experience and skill, and from this vantage point, higher opportunities for leadership either appear or can be created. These are 'higher' not in the sense that they are reserved for 'better' leaders but that they offer greater opportunity and possibility, often to help larger communities.

In the final chapter, we will revisit our personal influence and consider how we can adapt further to become effective at this higher level.

Although we can't be too specific about this 'higher' context, there are a few key differences compared to practice life, which will help us to be better prepared.

- Although some of the people with whom we work may be familiar to us, others may not be. In fact, there may be people who we meet for the first time in situations of significant influence, such as in board meetings. We may not have the advantages that come from an established *relationship*, but on the other hand, we have a chance to start with a clean sheet with some people.

- Even though there are differences between us, the people who work in a practice team have a shared *culture* born of their purpose and values. At a higher level, we may be working with communities that have quite different and at times, conflicting cultures. In addition if we are part of a *new community*, we may have an important role in bringing people together and shaping the identity and culture of the new group.

- We are unlikely to wield the same *authority* with the people with whom we work. Instead, we may well be working with people who have significant power that is independent from ours, and our influence, status and rank may be affected.

- People's *expectation* of us and our expectation of ourselves may be less clearly defined. Unlike being a doctor, nurse or manager, there might not be a rule book that says, for example, what a 'network lead' should be like.

- What about *knowledge*? In practice life, we may have a fairly thorough understanding of most aspects of our profession and business. This is unlikely to be the case in larger organisations where some areas of expertise and process may be opaque to us, or even kept from us.

- Leadership at a higher level is a more *public* affair. It attracts attention that we may not be used to and runs the risk of public shame, or just as toxic, public celebrity.

- We may face *ethical challenges* that are at odds with ourselves as people and as professionals. For example, we may face pressure to manage the message, giving it a spin that challenges our desire to be open and honest.

As we can begin to appreciate, the new context is unfamiliar, exposed, scary but exciting.

To gain influence, we may want to alter ourselves to fit the new context. That much is understandable. However, the world of greater opportunity is beset with the greatest temptations and the greatest risk of disconnection from our authentic selves. Power corrupts. No-one is exempt.

If there is an overarching message in this section, it is that we should be aware of the challenges, but do our best not to go too far and compromise who we are an our desire to do what we imagine is expected of us. Even more so than in our leadership journey thus far, it is by being true to ourselves and our values that we ultimately do the best for those we serve. That is why the final chapter of this book is a reminder to 'be yourself'.

This simple edict is, in practice, the hardest challenge we face and one that we can only rise to with the help of others. Every day we may fail, but every day we must try.

25

Be yourself

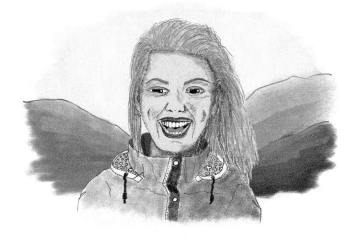

In this chapter, we will explore these questions:

- Why does it become even more important to be ourselves?
- How do we maintain our core values when we are in danger of being distanced from them?
- What could we do to help our colleagues to become more courageous?
- How does openness help us to develop new communities?
- Isn't being a clever politician, useful?
- How does competence also relate to standing back and to avoiding being exploited?
- How could we increase our informal influence when working with the powerful?
- What use could we make of people's resistance and friction?

Using our influence more effectively

In this chapter we will use the jigsaw pieces from Section 2 and focus on some of the personal attributes discussed there, illustrating their relevance and importance at this level. You may wish to refer back to these to appreciate how they have developed across our journey.

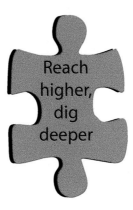

Dream on

As senior leaders, our higher visibility means that people look to us to articulate and reinforce our shared vision and values. At times, particularly when we are working across boundaries and developing new communities, we will need to revisit those values rather than assume them. Having a collective vision is not an administrative exercise but instead is a vital tool for keeping a new community on a shared track.

Therefore it becomes even more important that we remain connected to our deeper drives, such as the need to help people, be kind, enthuse, fight suffering or injustice and so on.

Case example

When Sunil became a senior GP commissioner, he felt that the organisations he was working with were like silos, focussing so much on their structure and boundaries that this distracted them from remaining connected to their core purpose and doing the right thing.

To remain connected, he did two things. First, he maintained his GP work one day a week. His consultations with his patients in particular, made him feel rooted in his purpose and gave him an outlet for

(Continued)

Case example (*Continued*)

his drive to help and to be kind. Second, he visited services every week, talking to providers and service users and hearing what people really thought. He felt that if he only heard about this from those people reporting to him, he would be told what they thought he wanted to hear and he would become disconnected from those whom he served.

This example also touches on the fact that in more senior positions, there is less opportunity to practice our chosen profession, which then creates a potential credibility gap with those who feel that we are no longer rooted, or even that we have sold out.

Everyone has their personal sense of what matters and connecting with others at this level is important. This especially includes those who are the most vocal *naysayers*. Consistently speaking up for what is important for the group, whilst respecting individual values and concerns, is noticed by others and helps to maintain our integrity.

Dig for victory

Let's consider two aspects here, health and courage. It's down to us, more so than down to others, to look after ourselves so that we can thrive. This may include taking care not to burn out. For this, we need to create sanctuaries like places or activities where we can restore our energy and maintain our optimism. The more senior we are the less time and encouragement we might have as there may be fewer colleagues who feel able or willing to enquire about our health and well-being, even if we are approachable people.

Case example

Anna, a regional practice nursing lead said, 'I have two families. At work, I have a very loyal group who are supportive of what I'm doing. I only need one or two people to be unconditionally supportive and these are people who know my journey and have seen me grow over the years. I know they have my back. Second, my real family are more important than ever as they help me with knowing right from wrong, and get me to use my moral compass and keep me on track'.

Regarding courage, we often talk about how we cope with adversity, but success can bring problems of its own that require us to be courageous.

Case example

A senior leader said, 'People will attack you, people react badly to success and the more success you have, the more attacks you get, especially from people and communities you thought had nothing to do with your enterprise. What keeps me going is the drive from within. I ask myself: Is this the right thing to do for people? This gives me courage and keeps me true to myself'.

Being bold encourages us to go beyond our authority. Boundaries are not permanent, they can be shifted. An important way of knowing where they lie is to test them and see where they bite back. This is obviously a risk, but making changes and asking for forgiveness rather than for permission, can help. However positive things will often happen, and going beyond the limitations imposed by ourselves or others, allows us to create new alliances that help with moving our efforts forward.

Case example

Greg, a part-time GP, was leading the city on reducing health inequalities. The city needed to increase physical activity to reduce obesity. He got a team together and told them, 'If we keep doing what we are doing, we won't crack the problem'. His bold question to the group was, 'What would we do if we had no organisational constraints?' This got people working beyond their assumed barriers and coming up with ways forward that were innovative and feasible.

Building on this, there is more we can do to nurture courageousness in the team. Here are some examples:

- Encourage the team to challenge the way we do things and identify processes that need to go. There are many protocols and procedures that although time-honoured are actually time-expired.
- Invite people from other communities, for example, the senior receptionist from a neighbouring practice, to use a fresh pair of eyes and ask 'Why?' and 'Why not?'. This can be particularly useful if facilitated well.

- Encourage innovation and risk-taking. Encourage people to run many small risks rather than one big one and bring together the information from these parallel experiments to plan what to do next.

- Reward risk-taking. For example, one organisation gives what it calls the 'turtle award' for people who, like the animal, stick their necks out in order to move forward.

- Have a plan, but be prepared to change it. No battle plan survives contact with the enemy and no work plan survives contact with the real world.

- Beyond making the current dysfunctional system more functional, encourage people to think afresh and challenge the system itself.

- Encourage people to raise issues and generate ideas across their borders rather than just within them. In this way, everyone is encouraged to *share* responsibility for problem-solving in the organisation.

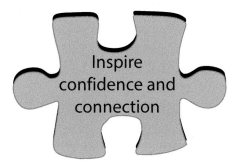

Compassion and courtesy

Treating people with kindness and unfailing courtesy keeps us on the best track. This becomes increasingly important as we work with people who don't know us either well or possibly, at all. These attributes are a good indicator of integrity, which is particularly important when there hasn't been the opportunity to form deeper relationships. Such relative strangers may know when and where we need assistance, even when we are not aware that we do, and our compassion and courtesy may motivate people to help us.

Being honest

When working across organisational boundaries, people judge each other quickly and on limited information. One of the most important things that people look for is whether they feel that we are being honest and genuine, and a significant but difficult façade to drop is that of 'knowing'.

As a senior GP representative on a trust board, Simon was new to the team. At his first meeting people were extensively using jargon, but rather than feeling embarrassed at his ignorance and just accepting this, Simon said, 'I'm sorry, I don't really know what is being said because I don't understand the jargon, but I'd like to give you my perspective. Please forgive me if I don't have the proper language'. People valued his honesty, warmed to his vulnerability and the chair responded by asking the group to use plain English. The ensuing discussion was much more fruitful, people later said.

So, just at the moment that we feel anxious because we are with people unfamiliar to us and wish to create a good impression and be accepted, we should remind ourselves not to pretend to be what we are not.

Being more we than I

Personal ambition and ego can drive some people to reach up and become leaders of high achievement. However, these qualities if overplayed can lead to self-orientation and narcissism, which act as a barrier that prevents others from wishing to strengthen their relationships with us. If we lose connection with people, we lose the possibility of enlisting their help at a larger scale.

Taking this concept beyond the individual, let us apply it to groups of people. As we become more experienced leaders, we usually find ourselves working with larger and more diverse communities. The tribes within these communities bring the strength of their individualism but also the ego that is part of their separate identities. By encouraging them to be more outward-orientated and collaborative, we can become more effective and expand our collective vision of ourselves, adding the strength of nationhood to the power of being tribes.

Being genuine and being open

Not pretending about ourselves and being open, especially about our vulnerabilities, helps people to connect strongly. We should show our genuine selves early and in appropriate settings.

Case example

Dilip is a regional director and part-time GP. When asked about where he felt vulnerable, he said:

Compared to practice life, in my senior role the people I mix with, particularly those outside the medical community, don't know me. This makes me feel vulnerable because they make inappropriate assumptions about me, especially my motives or behaviour. These are based on my new position and role, rather than any knowledge of me personally. Initially I was angry about this. Now I try sharing more and I've also stopped calling myself by my title of Regional Director, which I found just created fear and resentment. Instead, I introduce myself as a GP (which is the real 'me') and I get a much better response. This helps us work more effectively together, which is what it's all about.

'Being open' has other facets, including:

* ***Being open to new information.*** This means being more *observant*. One example is learning to 'read the room' and thereby quickly gauge new communities. By noticing how people behave, we can identify who supports and who stands in the way. This mental topography helps us to navigate a way through. Being a chair, as discussed in Chapter 20, is a good example of this.

* ***Being open to new possibilities*** and not allowing our assumptions to stand in the way. For example, being open about new roles and responsibilities such as not assuming that managers will always manage (and nothing else). Alternatively, being open involvement of other communities who want to play a part:

Case example

In the network community, the geographical area covered by the network became coterminous with other important services. The fire and rescue service heard about the importance of picking up on atrial fibrillation (AF) to prevent stroke. They volunteered to screen for AF during their routine assessments of people to whom they had been called. They were able to offer this to the network in a way that they would not have been able to do for individual practices. Their example showed that resources aren't always a barrier to doing things better.

- *Encouraging openness in others,* for example, bringing people together to work around common activities and tasks using a quality improvement mindset. This promotes mutual understanding and shared values as well as new ways of working that are less top-down.
- *Being open in the way we do things.* Applying this throughout the change cycle from openly discussing ideas, to weighing up the options and being open about the outcomes.

Integrity and politics

As we've previously noted, integrity is of absolute importance. However, politics can damage us, so how can we marry both?

First, do we need to? Small 'p' politics is about manipulating the environment to our advantage. This happens both by manipulating people and by manipulating the processes through which things happen.

We may think this doesn't apply to us, but is that the case? As leaders we are signed up to the art of using our influence effectively, so politics is not just unavoidable, it is necessary, not for accruing personal power but for helping our community.

However, politics can damage our integrity, so we need to be guided by our ethics so that we do the most good and the least harm. To accept that we will be political but at the same time aim to do it well, it helps to be:

- *Politically alert:* recognising the situations in which people are likely to be more manipulative than usual. This will be the case when the stakes are higher, for example, where the decisions are more important, people are competing for resources or individual advantage, more people are involved or affected or there is a higher degree of uncertainty.
- *Politically aware:* of the people and the processes. Ideally, we would like to build relationships, but in high-stakes situations there may not be the time or opportunity to do so and taking shortcuts can't be avoided. Some will behave with integrity and these people are potential allies.

    Others will behave in ways that might be described as clever, wily, devious, Machiavellian, etc. Examples include being self-orientated and seeking power, looking for weakness in others and exploiting this, playing to win and for others to lose, and so on. By being aware of the games people play, we can take steps not to be exploited by them.

    We can also become aware of who is aligned with whom, what people are driven by, where their lines in the sand lie, how they are likely to vote, and so on. Formal meetings as described in Chapter 20 are political environments; there is a clear parallel between what is described here and the vigilance that we use in chairing such meetings.

- *Politically astute:* in addition to getting to know the people and the connections between them, it's our business to get to understand the processes, how things get done, where influence and power lie, what levers or forms of persuasion exist or can be created and so on.

We are definitely not above temptation. By using our self-awareness and the guidance of those who know the importance of integrity, we can monitor our own game-playing and keep ourselves on track. We thereby do the best for our communities by using the processes of power well, not being naïve, treating people well and behaving with integrity. The last of these sounds straightforward but it will really test our courage if we are to be more open and honest than some people may advise.

Being competent

It can be helpful to know that it is a law of nature that initial turbulence will spontaneously settle itself over time. This means that in complex situations, competence can be as much about what we *don't* do, as well as what we do, for example, stepping back at times and allowing people to work through problems. In doing so, they improve their capabilities and we prevent our own burn-out.

As we become more open and people get more familiar with the way that we are tuned, we become more 'playable' or even 'seducible'. For example, people may know which buttons to press to get a reaction. They may offer inappropriate criticism or praise, both of which take our eye off the ball, or offer opportunities that channel our energy in a different direction.

This can threaten our competence, and to counter this we can develop a wider range of responses that make us both more adaptable and less predictable. Let's consider two examples of how we can broaden our responses.

First, if we had to block or re-channel a suggested course of action, we need not go about this in one predictable way. Instead, we could use a wider range of approaches such as the 'D's of declining, delaying, deferring, detouring, deterring, and denying.

Second, we could recognise our biases and learn to compensate for them and thereby avoid being predictable.

Case example

Laura, a clinical director said, 'I recognise that I like an underdog and sometimes I go too far in trying to help them. Because I have wider responsibilities as a senior leader, I can see that these actions are not always equitable, and I need to be seen to be fair to the wider community'.

Let's also consider the scope of competence. At a higher level of leadership influence, there is an expectation of competence in particular areas:

- We are expected to understand the organisation's structure, strategy, culture, finances and operations.
- Our 'conscientiousness' increasingly includes a concern for legality and regulations.
- As well as having an eye for the detail, we need the ability to step back and see the bigger picture. Putting the ability to notice the detail alongside the ability to visualise more broadly, helps us to see a picture emerging.
- We need to avoid trivial or inappropriate work, which might even be a refuge, so as to keep ourselves available for the more complex issues that need our expertise. The complexity of the problems we face, may mean that we need to take more 'time out' for thinking collectively.

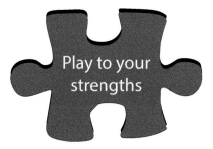

Being wise with our power

From our understanding of complexity, we know that the way forward can't be predetermined but has to be allowed to shape itself through adaptation. However, power can misdirect us, particularly when it tempts us to inappropriately control the situation. As an example, when we have worked significantly on an intervention, it may feel like 'ours', and this sense of ownership can make us place conditions on it, for instance, that it should go forward in particular ways. Instead, it could be more helpful to regard the intervention as having a life of its own. In this way we can reduce the bias that makes us see only what we want to see.

In addition, holding back from trying to take control stops us from micro-managing people, which helps them to develop their self-confidence and morale rather than become nervous or disengaged through our meddling.

Our power can give others confidence, so whilst 'letting go' we still need to be 'present', meaning that we are seen to be on top of things through being well-informed and through communicating well.

Although paradoxical, at a high level our official authority may have limited impact because we are dealing with other powerful people and our influence could be tempered by this. For leadership collectively, this is probably a good thing.

Because of this, our *informal* influence becomes even more important. This can be improved by:

- *Strengthening relationships* with people who have a significant stake in the issue
- *Delivering early wins,* which enhances our reputation for compe-tence and credibility as does
- *Under-promising and over-delivering* on our commitments
- *Making friends of those who have opposed us* in the past. Such people make extremely powerful allies and the example of rapprochement influences people widely and positively.
- *Talking up to power:* we can help people more powerful than our-selves by advising about areas of confusion and conflict. We can also advise about the reaction that they might anticipate with their pro-posals. Being informed and alerted (rather than being given advice) is appreciated by most effective leaders. Most importantly by help-ing them do the right thing, we can make sure that they don't over-look what's really important. Helping them helps us.

Case example

Jason was a new clinical director. At his first high-level meeting, which included a government minister, the group were talking about improving services but were overlooking the key issue of deprivation which Jason

(Continued)

knew to be vital. The meeting was extremely controlled through a tight agenda, so it was difficult to raise the issue. However, Jason was able to intervene effectively by showing respect and highlighting the positive messages that he had heard, pointing out what was missing and why this was important. This went down well, and his points were noted.

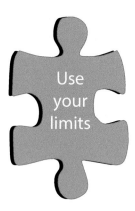

Seeing our limits as opportunities

We are limited in a number of dimensions that are relevant here. We are limited:

- In the range of ability within the team, and need to nurture this
- By our biases, and need to knowingly challenge our assumptions and thereby engage a broader range of people
- By the desire for harmony, and need to make use of diversity
- By our shelf-life and our usefulness to the team, and need to plan for succession

We will explore each of these here.

Through greater understanding of the need for strong and capable teams, along with greater power to create opportunities, we can increasingly:

- ***Identify and unleash talent.*** Our support won't be in the form of micromanaging but more along the lines of hand-holding, coaching, mentorship and noticing and valuing what people do.

- *Identify the energy.* Rather than just using our rational minds, as experienced leaders we also learn to feel for the energy. Whenever there is a choice that could involve a change in direction of travel, we can get a sense where interest lies, and where it doesn't. Interest is another word for positive energy. We can then harness the energy where the interest lies and where the motivation actually is, rather than where our biases make us believe it should be. If we can overcome our frustrations and be more flexible, we can use this as the starting point for quality improvement through experimentation and evaluation.

- *Direct the energy usefully.* Because of our biases, people's interest could be viewed as positive or negative, for or against. However we can learn to avoid these limiting categorisations, and instead have the mindset that *all* energy is potentially useful. Our goal then becomes to harness and direct it, and this reduces our tendency to avoid conflict and resistance or fear those who stand in the way. Instead, we can engage with such people more productively. For example, by helping them to use the power that they are feeding into their resistance and redirect it into such things as problem-solving or new tasks and opportunities.

Case example

Ollie, a medical director for the city, needed to appoint clinical leads from each neighbourhood of local practices. In one area no one wanted to lead, but one of the doctors was consistently vocal, although always negatively so. Ollie spoke to her and helped her to see that her passion and drive made her stand out. He showed her that there had been discussions at a higher level initiated by her challenges, that had led to changes. He helped her see that leadership was not about popularity but about caring, which she clearly did. Having thought about this, she was persuaded to take the post and later was successful as an advocate for her community.

- *Harness diversity.* Diversity is painted in a positive light; this is a good thing because it is a source of our adaptability. However it is not necessarily comfortable, because this adaptability arises from our disagreement and friction. As experienced leaders, we not only use diversity but also deliberately bring it into the team, perhaps through recruitment, recognising that diversity and disharmony will go hand-in-hand. Of course, this is only wise if we have the skills to manage diversity well. If we don't, we may quickly blamed for the disruption that it causes.

- ***Make ourselves dispensable.*** If this is planned well so that people have sufficient skills and confidence to problem-solve and take action, then removing ourselves from the front line is not so much abdication, as empowerment. Through developing individuals, augmented by on-the-job debriefing, we build leadership capacity. In such ways, we can move our organisation from being top-down and leader-led, to becoming more horizontal and leader-full.

Case example

Helen enabled her team by encouraging others to chair meetings that she attended. She didn't speak but was ready to intervene if needed. She also took certain tasks so far and then handed over for someone else to complete, under her supervision. Her colleagues gained from her support and mentorship and she also learned to let go and to avoid saying that she would have done things a different way.

Over the stile

As we reach the final stile of this book, we cannot predict or guide where your journey will lead beyond it. Looking back, we hope that this exploration has enriched your understanding of leadership. More importantly, looking forward we hope that it inspires you to help others make *their* difference. If it does, then our hike together has been worthwhile, and we are with you in spirit as your adventure takes you in a new direction.

Bibliography

Barlow, J. & Moller, C. (2008). *A Complaint Is a Gift: Recovering Customer Loyalty When Things Go Wrong* (2nd ed.). Berrett-Koehler Publishers.

Bass, B. & Riggio, R. (2006). *Transformational Leadership* (2nd ed.). Mahwah, NJ: Lawrence Erlbaum Associates.

Bate, P. (2014). *Context Is Everything: In Perspectives in Context*. London, UK: The Health Foundation. Available at http://health.org.uk/publications/perspectives-on-context/

Berne, E. (1964). *Games People Play: The Psychology of Human Relationships*. New York: Ballantine Books.

Berwick, D. (2013). *A Promise to Learn – A Commitment to Act: Improving the Safety of Patients in England*. London, UK: Department of Health and Social Care.

Binney, G., Wilke, G., & Williams, C. (2005). *Living Leadership: A Practical Guide for Ordinary Heroes*. London, UK: Prentice Hall.

Bjergegaard, M. & Popa, C. (2016). *How to Be a Leader*. Macmillan. ISBN: 978-1-447293279.

Bowie, P. et al. (2016). Enhancing the effectiveness of significant event analysis: Exploring personal impact and applying systems thinking in primary care. *Journal of Continuing Education in the Health Professions* 36, doi:10.1097/CEH.0000000000000098.

Bridges, W. (2017). *Managing Transitions: Making the Most of Change* (4th ed.). London, UK: Nicholas Brealey Publishing. ISBN-10: 1473664500.

Brown, A. (2014). *The Myth of the Strong Leader*. Vintage. ISBN: 9780099554851.

Brown, B. (2012). *Daring Greatly*. Penguin Random House UK. ISBN: 978-0-241-25740-1.

Buckingham, M. & Clifton, D. (2001). *Now, Discover Your Strengths*. The Gallup Organization. ISBN: 1-4165-0265-3.

Bushe, G.R. & Marshak, R. (2015). *Dialogic Organization Development: The Theory and Practice of Transformational Change*. Berrett-Koehler Publishers. ISBN: 978-1-62656-404-6.

Carey, R.G. & Lloyd, R.C. (1995). *Measuring Quality Improvement in Healthcare*. New York, NY: ASQ Quality Press.

Committee on Quality of Health Care in America. (2001). *Crossing the Quality Chasm: A New Health System for the 21st Century*. Washington, DC: National Academy Press.

Covey, S.R. (2004). *The 7 Habits of Highly Effective People: Powerful Lessons in Personal Change*. London, UK: Simon & Schuster.

Coyle, D. (2018). *The Culture Code: The Secrets of Highly Successful Groups*. Banton Books. ISBN: 978-1-52479709-6.

Cunliffe, A. (2014). *A Very Short, Fairly Interesting and Reasonably Cheap Book about Management*. Sage Publications. ISBN: 97814 4627 3500.

Darzi, A. (2008). *High Quality Care for All*. London, UK: Department of Health.

Davis, J. (2016). *The Greats on Leadership: Classic Wisdom for Modern Managers*. Nicholas Brearley Publishing. ISBN: 978-1-85788-648-1.

Diamond, J. (2016). *Power: A User's Guide*. Belly Song Press. ISBN: 978-0-0996 6603-0-3.

Downey, M. (2003). *Effective Coaching* (3rd ed.). Texere Publishing.

Gillam, S. & Siriwardena, A.N. (2014). *Quality Improvement in Primary Care: The Essential Guide*. London, UK: Radcliffe.

Grint, K. (2005). Problems, problems, problems: The social construction of leadership. *Human Relations* 58(11), 1467–1494.

Health Improvement Scotland. (2012). Safequest safety climate survey. Available at http://www.healthcareimprovementscotland.org/our_work/patient_safety/spsp_primary_care_resources/safety_climate_survey.aspx

Heifetz, R., Grashow, A., & Linsky, M. (2009). *The Practice of Adaptive Leadership*. Harvard Business Review Press. ISBN: 978-14221-0576-4.

Heron, J. (1989). *Six Category Intervention*. Surrey, UK: University of Surrey.

Hersey, P. & Blanchard, K.H. (2000). *Management of Organizational Behaviour: Utilizing Human Resources*. Classiques Hachette. ISBN: 9780132617697.

Hogan, C. (2003). *Practical Facilitation: A Toolkit of Techniques*. London, UK: Kogan Page.

Hughes, R., Ginnett, R., & Curphy, G. (2002). *Leadership: Enhancing the Lessons of Experience*. McGraw-Hill Higher Education. ISBN: 0-07-244529-7.

Ishikawa, K. (1968). *Guide to Quality Control*. Tokyo: JUSE.

Issacs, W. (1999). *Dialogue and the Art of Thinking Together*. New York: Doubleday.

Kahane, A. (2017). *Collaborating with the Enemy*. Berrett-Koehler Publishers. ISBN: 9781626568228.

Kelley, R. (1992). *The Power of Followership*. Bantam Dell.

Kotter, J. (2012). *Leading Change*. Harvard Business Review. ISBN-10: 9781422186435.

Ladkin, L. (2010). *Rethinking Leadership: A New Look at Old Leadership Questions.* MPG Books Group UK. ISBN: 9781847209351.

Langley, G.J. et al. (2009). *The Improvement Guide: A Practical Approach to Enhancing Organizational Performance* (2nd ed.). San Francisco, CA: Jossey-Bass. ISBN: 978-0-470-19241-2.

Lewis, S., Passmore, J., & Cantore, S. (2011). *Appreciative Inquiry for Change Management: Using AI to Facilitate Organizational Development.* London, UK: Kogan-Page.

Mullins, C. & Constable, G. (2007). *Leadership and Team Building in the Primary Care.* London, UK: Radcliffe. ISBN: 978-1-84619-105-3.

NHS England. *National GP Patient Survey.* https://www.gp-patient.co.uk/

NHS Improvement. Root Cause Analysis – Using 5 Whys. https://improvement. nhs.uk/documents/2156/root-cause-analysis-five-whys.pdf 9/12/2019

On Leadership. (2011). Harvard Business Review Press. ISBN: 978-1-4221-5797-8.

Owen, J. (2011). *How to Lead.* Pearson. ISBN: 978-0-273-75961-4.

Pearson, C. (2012). *The Transforming Leader.* Thomson Press. ISBN: 978-1-60994-765-1.

Pendleton, D. & Furnham, A. (2012). *Leadership: All You Need to Know.* Basingstoke, UK: Palgrave Macmillan. ISBN: 978-0-230-31945-5.

Phillips, A. (2013). *Developing Leadership Skills for Health and Social Care Professionals.* Radcliffe. ISBN: 978-1-84619-883-0.

Rotter, J.B. (1966). Generalized expectancies for internal versus external control of reinforcement. *Psychological Monographs: General and Applied* 80, 1–28. doi:10.1037/h0092976.

Scharmer, O. (2016). *Theory U: Leading from the Future as It Emerges* (2nd ed.). Dreamscape Media. ISBN-13: 978-1626567986.

Schein, E.H. (2010). *Organizational Culture and Leadership* (4th ed.). San Francisco, CA: Jossey-Bass.

Senior, B. (2002). *Organizational Change.* Pearson. ISBN: 0-1273-65153-6.

Sinek, S. (2011). *Start with Why: How Great Leaders Inspire Everyone to Take Action.* London, UK: Penguin. ISBN-10: 9780241958223.

Spurgeon, P. & Clark, J. (2018). *Medical Leadership: The Key to Medical Engagement and Effective Organisations.* CRC Press. ISBN: 978-1-78523-161-2.

Stacey, R. (2012). *The Tools and Techniques of Leadership and Management: Meeting the Challenge of Complexity.* London, UK: Routledge.

Suderman, J. *Leading Globally: Understanding Cultural Assertiveness.* Available at http://jeffsuderman.com/leading-globally-understanding-cultural-assertiveness

West, M.A. (2012). *Effective Teamwork: Practical Lessons from Organisational Research* (3rd ed.). John Wiley & Sons and the British Psychological Society. ISBN: 978-0-470-97497-1.

Wiggins, L. & Hunter, H. (2016). *Relational Change: The Art and Practice of Changing Organizations.* Bloomsbury Business.

Wiseman, L. (2010). *Multipliers.* HarperCollins.

Index